the joy of
YOGA

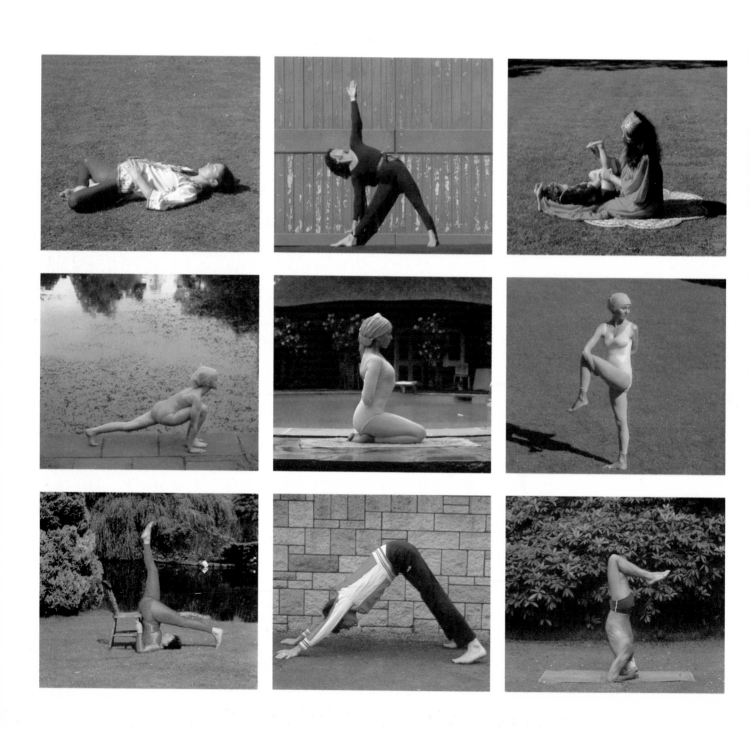

the joy of
YOGA

Rosalind Widdowson

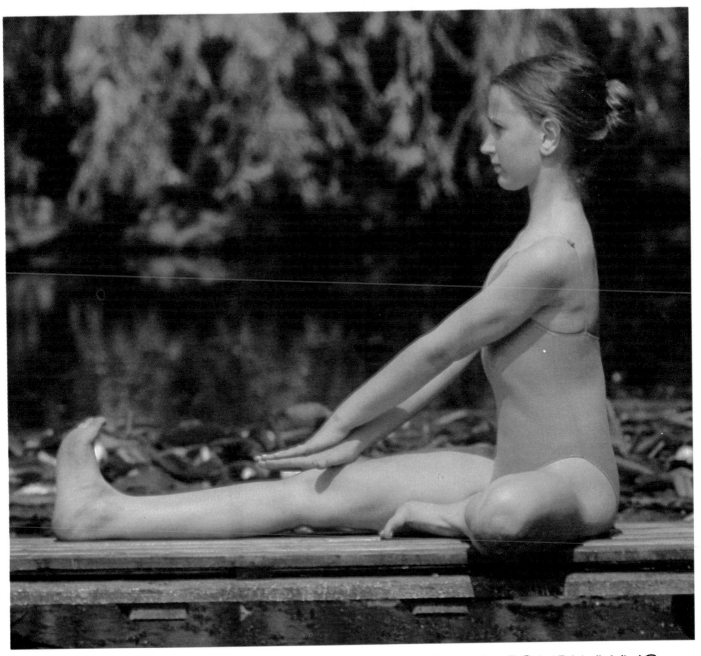

A DOLPHIN BOOK DOUBLEDAY & COMPANY INC.
Garden City, New York, 1983

Acknowledgments

The author and publishers would like to make special thanks to the following, who helped to make this book possible: Susan and Elizabeth Allen, Iris Baggot, Lisa Beaman, Mr and Mrs G. Clancey, Mary Davies, Bridgette Downing, Sue Delahay, Pam Griffith, Shawn Hawkins, Dexter Hunt, Jean Oddy, Helena Oliver, Ka Price, Myli and Zoë Philips, Harry Siviter, Jean Smith, Joanne Talbot, Tony Taylor, Linda Walker, Helen Tate, Tibort, Sarah Wakefield, Eileen Westly, Mark Widdowson, Briar Wilkinson, Halgey Sports and Leisure Limited of Hagley, Worcestershire, and Nigel Snowdon Associates of Bromley, Kent, who took the photographs.

A Dolphin Book
First published in USA in 1983
by Doubleday & Company, Inc.
Garden City, New York

Library of Congress Cataloging in Publication Data

Widdowson, Rosalind.
  The joy of yoga.

  Includes index.
  1. Yoga, Hatha. I. Title.
RA781.7.W53 1983   613.7'046   82-45874
ISBN 0-385-19006-9

Printed in Italy

Contents

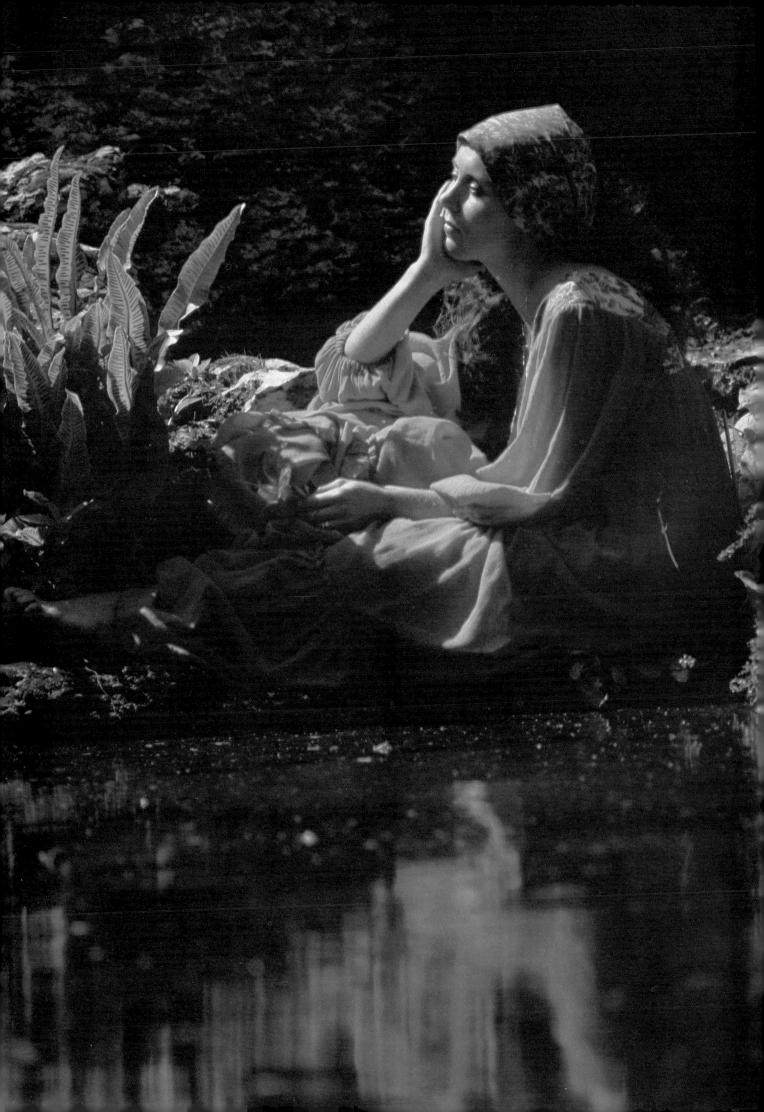

Introduction

I began Yoga at the age of four. Exercise has been a part of my life ever since.

Technique often seems difficult, unpleasant, and perhaps even a little humiliating. But many can vouch for the way Yoga has brought about a real and profound change in personal outlook. It represents a very direct approach to personal difficulties and undesirable feelings and habits. In time it can make life less harsh, and the people you meet in everyday life seem much more pleasant. The real change, of course, is in yourself: you are beginning to find inner peace and in turn, like a mirror, reflect tranquillity outwards. By helping yourself, you can help your fellow human beings.

Practise with patience and perseverance, rather than expecting spectacular results immediately. We are all, in fact, our own hardest critics and teachers. Be kind to yourself. Take one step at a time. Do not look continually for the goal; think of the means by which it may be achieved. Gradually the bonds of even your worst habits will loosen.

Yoga is no religion. It's a philosophy for life and, as such, it can enhance religious beliefs or perhaps persuade you to allow your own particular god to enter your awakened soul.

I do not profess to be a 'qualified' philosopher. Philosophy is not, I think, an intellectual science but the very act of living life to the full. Here are some of the simple beliefs that Yoga has taught me:

Balance Everyone has one side which is better than the other. Think of the movie star who always insists on being photographed on his or her 'best' side. Yoga helps you to perfect a harmonious control between the right and left sides of yourself by searching within to find and strengthen the weaknesses in body, mind, and spirit. By uniting yourself, you feel a greater unity with your fellow human beings.

Discipline All creative drive and purity must come from within. Find a purpose. See it clearly and work towards it. You have a natural inner strength. Try to remember this through the good and bad times, harnessing this inner energy.

Freedom Enjoy all you do. That way you help to free yourself from self-consciousness.

Intelligence Thought alone does not necessarily solve problems, but observation and acting upon natural instincts or intuition without undue delay can.

Love Personal experience of suffering can provide you with inner strength and greater love and compassion for others.

Positiveness Try to cancel all negative thoughts and actions with a positive approach to life. Live in the present, thinking of problems as possible opportunities and acting upon them.

Through many years of really enjoying Yoga I have met lots of interesting and inspiring people, all of whom have been as enthusiastic as I am about the new potentials which the practice of Yoga seems to release. My own innermost artistic talents might have lain dormant had I not been lucky enough to study this fascinating subject. My only wish is that this book may help you in a similar way.

Ros Widdowson.

The Widdowson Yoga, Health and Beauty Centres, Rock, Worcestershire, England.

Before you begin

Health precautions

If you have any serious health problems, ask your doctor whether or not you should do regular exercise. It's a sensible precaution to take anyway if you're over 35 and have grown lazy about taking exercise. Many doctors are now aware of the value of Yoga and frequently recommend it for people suffering the effects of stress and tension or for those recovering from broken or severely strained limbs.

There are some temporary and permanent health conditions which make it sensible to avoid *some* exercises. Check the following list and refer back to it from time to time.

Damaged limbs If you have deformed or damaged limbs, never strain to attain a posture. Your body will move when it is ready.

High blood pressure/Heart conditions/Weak eye capillaries/Detached retina Do not do the inverted (or upside down) exercises.

Hearing weakness Do not be alarmed if your balancing poses are not what you would like them to be. Try practising with a chair or against a wall to gain confidence. Be careful when practising the backward movements: they may need some gentle assistance.

Varicose veins Avoid holding the cross-legged or sitting-on-feet poses as these restrict the flow of blood through the veins. Include stretching and relaxing leg movements in your daily programme.

Hernias All back-bending movements should be avoided or taken only to a very slight stretch.

Menstruation If having a heavy period, avoid inverted postures like the Headstand or Shoulder Stand. Breathing exercises with stomach contractions or uplifts should also be avoided. The Plough and Shoulder Stand will, with regular practice, give relief to painful periods.

Pregnancy Relaxation and meditation can be practised all the way through your pregnancy. Apart from avoiding the obvious inverted movements mentioned for menstruation, overhead arm movements should also not be held for too long.

Just one more warning before I leave the subject of health precautions and that's about **Dizziness**. As with all exercises, if you feel any discomfort or dizziness, stop, lie down and relax for a few minutes before continuing. It is quite common to feel a slight choking sensation when first learning to do the Plough or Shoulder Stand. This is due to the increased blood supply gained from the inverted position, and to the gentle pressure to the throat and thyroid region. Try to relax the throat by gentle swallowing and, if necessary, breathe through the mouth to your own natural rhythm. If these choking sensations continue, you should get someone to help you improve your technique or avoid the exercise as it may not be suitable to your general physical make-up.

Preparing for Yoga

Choose, if possible, a quiet, well-ventilated room in which to practise. Ideally, it should be somewhere you know you won't be interrupted and a place you can use for every session.

Do not practise on a full stomach. Allow at least 3–4 hours after a meal before you start. This prevents unnecessary cramp and discomfort. Try not to eat immediately after a practice session either; an interval of half an hour makes a great deal of difference to your general sense of well-being.

Wear loose-fitting garments. The important thing is to avoid restrictive clothing, such as belts or waist bands. Most people now wear all-in-one leotards or track suits. Bare feet are essential to help improve the circulation of blood to the feet and keep control of the balancing movements.

Progress: or when can I do the Lotus?

Begin by spending several weeks on the section on Relaxation and Breathing which follows (see page 15). Slowly and without strain, introduce the simple stretching exercises described in that section. If you venture no further, you will already have an exercise programme which makes a real contribution to the elimination of tension.

Later use the problem-solving section: pages 19–67. There you'll find exercise schedules tailored to suit a great variety of conditions, ages and requirements.

Later still you may find the section on Yogarhythm on pages 69 to 73 rewarding. Using my classical-dance training, I have been able to choreograph all the Yoga exercises I have learnt into simple sequences which make it easier to remember them. Performed to a musical accompaniment, sequences like this can be an enjoyable, modern way to practise the ancient art of Yoga.

Whichever way you choose to use this book, remember that though these exercises may look static, they are, in fact, dynamic. Your mind, body and spirit should be totally involved in stretching to the maximum without unnecessary strain, taking each movement through all its preparatory stages before attempting the final dynamic pose.

In time you must try to find your own dynamic pose, the one which best suits both your temperament and your general way of life. Once found, you should practise it daily, holding it in perfect stillness to slow the racing mind and recharge the system.

Practise with patience and perseverance, remembering that progress varies according to the individual's general fitness, age, or specific disabilities. There is no need to compare your progress with that of others. The important point to remember is that *quality* of movement is your goal. Simply do the best you can; *enjoy* your exercises. It doesn't matter if for weeks, or months, you can't get further than stage 2 in an 8-part exercise without strain. Forget the other six parts and concentrate on doing the first two really well. In a while you'll find that stage 3 isn't so difficult after all, and then stage 4. . . .

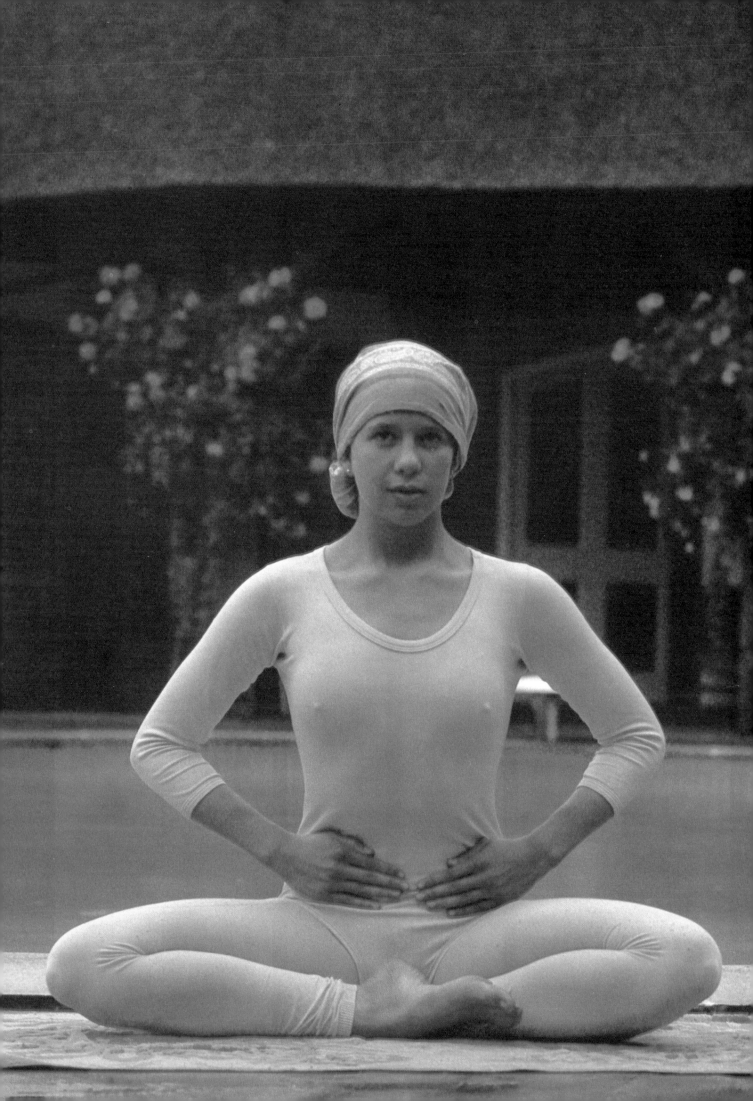

Breathing and Relaxation

The dangers of stress

Many leading physicians are now convinced that ailments such as mental illness, cancer, multiple sclerosis, arthritis, peptic ulcers, blood pressure, heart disease and premature ageing are caused by an inability to cope with stress.

Understanding and coping with stress is an important part of understanding and preventing ill health.

The key to lasting health and beauty is to use stress to your advantage. We all need stress to live. Without physical and mental challenges our bodies become feeble and we lose the excitement of enthusiastic living.

The secret of controlling stress is to create a balanced way of living. How is this done? By cultivating a programme of moderation in drinking, adequate sleep, regular balanced meals, daily exercise, and proper relaxation. I'll be talking about Yoga exercise and diet later, but I want to begin with the most vital of all subjects – relaxation and breathing.

How can I relax?

Everyone needs to relax mind and body at least once during the day: busy housewife, business executive, manual worker, invalid, old and young alike. Try to spare just a few minutes at the same time every day. A short period of complete relaxation from daily routine will bring renewed vigour to enjoy the rest of your day.

Most of us have forgotten the art of relaxation. We knew it instinctively as babies and forgot it as the pressures and pace of modern living worked upon us. Many people equate relaxation with play. 'Oh, yes,' they declare. 'We had a really relaxing holiday.' And then reel off a list of activities – sightseeing, shopping, meeting friends. Their leisure time has obviously been scheduled just as closely as their work time.

What I mean by relaxation is a deep release from all the tensions of your life by the re-centring of yourself *in* yourself. We spend so much of our lives being what other people want us to be, doing what is expected of us. It is easy to lose the sense of our own separate and special identity. Only by uniting the elements of ourselves in peace can we find real harmony. Learning to relax is an important step along that route. Here is my own formula for relaxation.

Lie on the ground, flat on your back, with your legs 30–60cm (1–2ft) apart, your arms lying free from the sides of your body, the fingers curling naturally. Gently close your eyes. You are lying in what is known as the **Resting Pose** (or Corpse Pose). Breathe to your own natural rhythm and surrender to relaxation by releasing your limbs from physical tensions thinking:

> My feet relax outwards.
> My ankles are relaxed.
> My knees are really relaxed.
> My thighs are beautifully relaxed.
> My hips relax.

> My stomach is relaxed.
> My ribs and chest expand freely and relax.
> My shoulders relax downwards and outwards.
> My arms relax through to each fingertip and my fingers curl naturally.
> My scalp feels relaxed, releasing the tensions of the day through every hair follicle.
> My face is beautifully relaxed.
> My eyes are sinking, sinking into the depths of relaxation.
> Lines of worry are soothed away.
> My lips gently open.
> My jaws are free, allowing my breath to flow naturally to every neglected part of my body.
> With my body and mind really relaxed, I rest.

Perform this routine gently and with patience, and even after a week of daily practice you will be feeling its benefits.

I know many people find it difficult to relax to order or even to understand what is meant by relaxation. I think it is best described as a sense that your body has spread and lengthened to feel light and free. For anyone who has difficulties I suggest the technique of stretching and letting go. Stretch your feet and then let that tension go. Feel it seeping away. Do the same with your knees and so on. Remember the feeling as the tension leaves your limbs. That is what you are aiming for as you relax.

Learning to breathe the Yoga way

Once you have begun to relax from the pressures of day-to-day life, you will become more aware of your breathing rhythms. Most of the time you probably breathe fairly rapidly and shallowly. Notice how, as you lie in the Resting Pose, practising relaxation, your breathing rate seems to slow and grow deeper. Think about occasions when you've been worried or upset. Doesn't your breathing become fast and uneven?

Your breathing rhythms are obviously linked to your state of mind. When you are calm, you breathe steadily; when you are disturbed, breathing becomes disjointed. If you still need convincing, remember the traditional advice to take three deep breaths before starting a difficult task. Or breathe really rapidly for a minute and see how uneasy you begin to feel.

If it is this easy to control your emotions, then there must be much to gain from learning to breathe in a rhythmic way. It's a stage on the route to personal harmony.

We usually leave everyday breathing to haphazard control by the body's automatic reflexes and the unconscious mind. Yoga breathing aims to bring the whole breathing system under conscious control. We do it by becoming aware of the body mechanisms involved and deliberately modifying the rhythm and force of our breathing.

The Complete Breath

The simplest of the Yoga breathing exercises is the **Complete Breath**. Don't confuse complete breath with deep breath. A Complete Breath involves all the stale air being forced out of your lungs before fresh air is drawn in, and the whole of your torso being free to participate in the breath.

Many of us suffer from a form of 'frozen torso', trying to breathe without moving the ribs or abdomen properly. Take a look at the two diagrams which show what happens when

is regular practice which helps you make changes in yourself. The rule about whether you have done enough is simple. If you begin to feel strained, then it is time to stop.

I'll begin with three preliminary exercises which help you to *place* your breathing – in the upper chest, the ribcage, and the abdomen. When you're confident you can perform these, try the Complete Breath.

Incidentally, unless otherwise stated, all the Yoga breathing exercises in this book require you to breathe through the nose. So it's a good idea to blow it carefully before beginning.

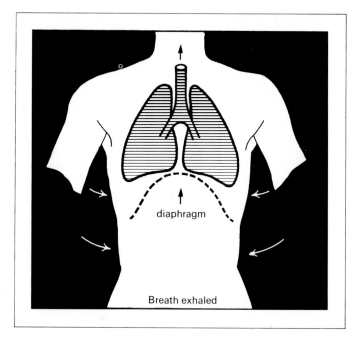

Note the diaphragm movement

Breath inhaled

diaphragm

Breath exhaled

you take the Complete Breath. It is the diaphragm, the sheet of muscle separating chest from abdomen, which is the controlling agent.

> **Diaphragm contracts**, moving **down**, and the entire ribcage expands outwards and upwards as air rushes in to expand the lower, middle and upper parts of the lungs.
> **Diaphragm relaxes**, coming **up**, and carbon dioxide is expelled from the lungs as the ribcage contracts downwards.

It is best to begin practising the Complete Breath by lying on the ground on your back with your knees bent. That way you can really feel what happens to your ribs and diaphragm when you breathe. Later, once you understand the technique, it can also be practised sitting or standing, and you'll be able to take a few Complete Breaths at any time and almost anywhere it suits you.

All Yoga breathing exercises are powerful stuff. Perform them for brief periods but regularly, every day if possible. It

Upper chest Place palms on upper chest, fingertips touching. *Exhale*, emptying your lungs completely. *Inhale* slowly, pushing fingertips apart until the chest can expand no more. *Exhale* in one continuous movement, chest contracting until fingertips again touch.

Ribcage Rest palms on lower ribcage, fingertips touching, and *exhale* to empty lungs. *Inhale* slowly, expanding ribs and pushing hands apart. *Exhale*, slowly relaxing muscles between ribs.

Abdomen Place palms on stomach and *exhale* to empty lungs. Slowly *inhale*, contracting diaphragm. Although you can't feel the diaphragm directly, you can sense pressure on the muscles at the top of the stomach which the diaphragm displaces as it moves down. *Exhale* smoothly, feeling muscles relax as diaphragm relaxes upwards.

Complete Breath : Lying Down Begin with palms resting on stomach and *exhale* to empty lungs. *Inhale*

slowly, sliding hands upwards while diaphragm moves down (exerting pressure on stomach muscles) and ribcage expands outwards and upwards as lungs fill with air. *Exhale*, relaxing diaphragm and sliding hands back down to stomach as carbon dioxide is expelled. Repeat the complete movement with your arms resting by your sides.

Now, keeping your arms by your sides, try breathing the Complete Breath to your own **natural rhythm**. This means that you observe your own breathing reflex and breathe only when it demands. *Exhale* and make no attempt to *inhale* until your body demands it. Then *inhale* really deeply. *Exhale* again only when your body tells you to. You'll find your body pauses for longer when your lungs are empty than when they are full. Make no attempt to force your breathing into any specific pattern. Concentrate on making sure all of the air goes out of your lungs, and they will refill entirely automatically.

This is natural breathing and it is the pattern of breathing you should use when you are holding any completed Yoga posture unless instructed otherwise. The basic rule for linking breathing to posture is as follows:

> *exhale* as you bend
> *natural breathing* as you hold a posture
> *inhale* as you straighten up

Certain forms of Yoga demand more precisely controlled patterns of breathing but this basic rule holds good for almost all the postures.

Counting the breath is the next step in control. Begin with a regular pattern of 1–5 counts (each count equals 1 second), gradually increasing the count at your own pace. Repeat your maximum count 2–3 times. The length of time taken over the exercise will vary from one person to another, but try to keep to the same length of time by perhaps cutting down on the number of times you repeat the exercise as you lengthen your count. Once you have learnt the basic technique, try to practise with your eyes closed, pinpointing your mind on the in and out flow of breath. As you take air into your lungs, think of the breath of life streaming freely into your body. As you breathe out, think of all the impurities and tensions flowing away.

Yoga offers a wide variety of other breathing patterns and techniques. You'll find some elsewhere in this book, among them the Alternate Nostril Breath with its vital calming properties. Certain techniques will require you to hold the breath either in or out. Don't attempt any of these until you feel really confident about the Complete Breath. As always, the important thing is the *quality* of your breathing, not the rate of progress.

The Complete Breath alone has many benefits to offer: it increases vitality, tones up the nervous system, purifies the blood, aids digestion, and strengthens the whole chest.

When to practise

Breathing exercises are best practised first thing you get up, before breakfast, or before retiring to bed. Ideally 3–4 hours should have elapsed since your last meal and half an hour since your last drink. All the other points about preparing for Yoga mentioned on page 13 apply here too.

Checklist for Yoga breathing

Aim for brief, regular practice
Ideal time: getting up and going to bed
Normal rule: *exhale* to bend, *natural breathing* to hold, *inhale* to straighten
Keep your eyes closed to centre your concentration.
Increase breath count very gradually
Relax in Resting Pose

Stretch and Relax

Now you've thought about relaxation and breathing, and familiarized yourself with two very basic and important techniques, it's time to begin exercising that body of yours.

What follows is simply a series of simple stretches. These are very basic movements, fundamental principles (if you like) that underlie many of the Yoga exercises you'll learn later. If you can spend some weeks on these, coupled with your breathing and relaxation techniques, you'll approach the exercise schedules that follow already feeling fitter and looking better. And you'll be in that more relaxed state in which real personal growth can occur.

Stretch: 1 Lie on your stomach, straight arms apart and forward, palms downwards, legs comfortably apart and forehead to ground. *Inhale* 1–5, contracting torso, arching backwards, and raising stretched arms and legs. Hold maximum position for 1–5 counts. *Exhale* 1–5, relaxing torso, legs and arms to ground, head to side, elbows slightly bent.

2 Roll over onto back, arms still over head, palms uppermost, legs apart. *Inhale* 1–5, contracting torso up off ground to balance on shoulders and heels with feet arched and arms stretched. Hold for 1–5. *Exhale* 1–5, relaxing to ground.

3 Bring arms down to sides and, still lying on back, bend knees. *Inhale* 1–5, raising and straightening legs. Slide hands down stretched legs to arched feet. Hold maximum position for 1–5. *Exhale* 1–5, relaxing to starting position. Variation: raise torso and legs up to balanced 'V' position.

4 From a seated position, with legs straight and hands on upper thighs, *inhale* 1–5. *Exhale* 1–5, sliding hands forward and down stretched legs and arched feet. Hold maximum position for 1–5. *Inhale* to upright position and *exhale*.

Repeat each exercise 1–5 times. Introduce variations by: (1) keeping legs and arms together, and (2) flexing toes up.

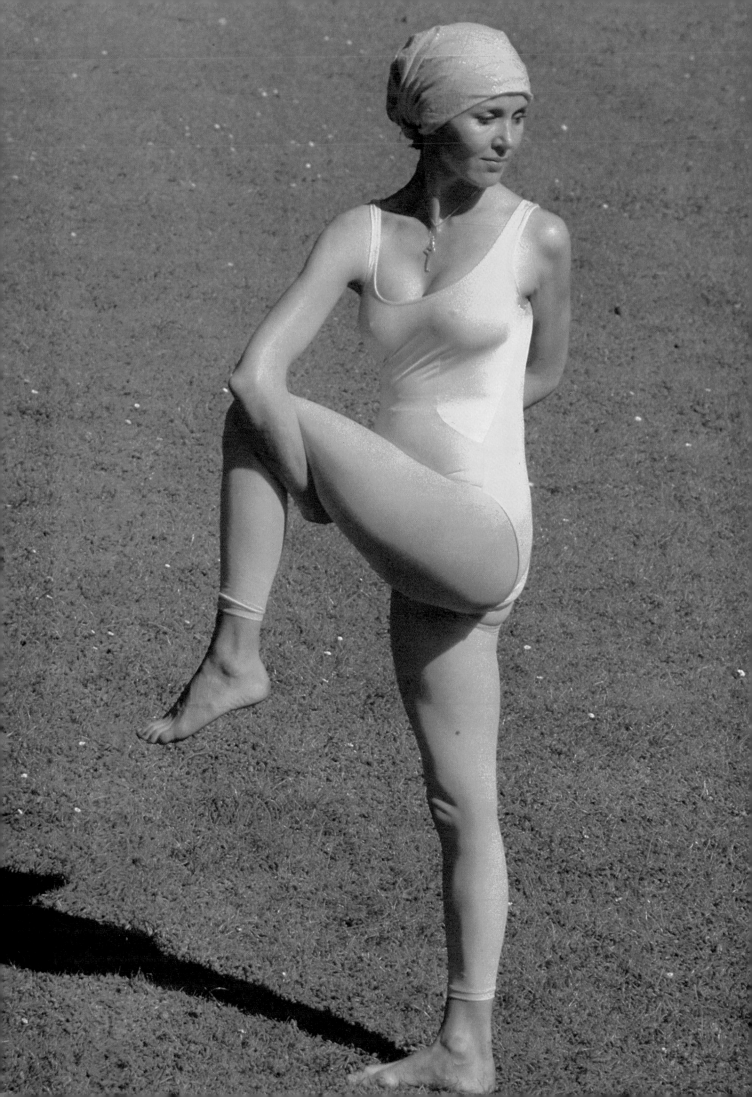

Pressures of Modern Living
Overwork

The problem It is very easy to overwork. Sometimes when life looks bleak, we use work like a drug. Sometimes we try to compensate for general ineffectiveness.

The solution The secret is to find the right balance between work and play. The practice of Yoga increases the mental and spiritual energy we need to discover and continually exercise that balance. If you bring total awareness to your Yoga sessions, you will soon begin to sense a freshness in your approach to life.

As mentioned on page 13, the aim of every Yoga student should be to find his or her own dynamic pose. Turn to the Yogarhythm section which begins on page 69 and try practising those sequences. It's possible you'll come across your dynamic pose there. If not, look through the rest of the book and experiment for yourself. The simple exercise below is a preliminary relaxation to your own dynamic pose.

Breathing pattern Normal (see page 17). No hold for Complete Breath.

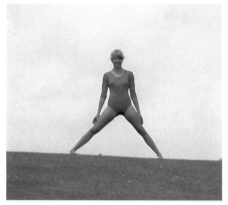

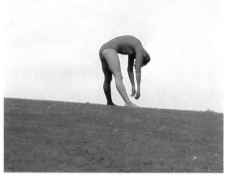

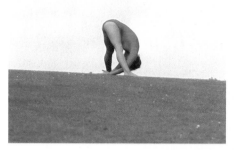

Rag Doll: 1 Stand with legs 60–90cm (2–3ft) apart. *Inhale* deeply, stretching spine upwards.

2 *Exhale* slowly, relaxing body forward from head to pelvis with arms hanging free.

3 Continue relaxation to farthest possible position, ideally with arms hanging between straight legs.

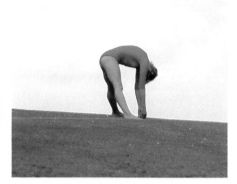

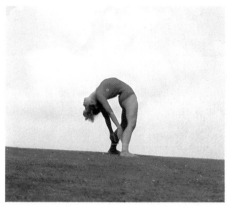

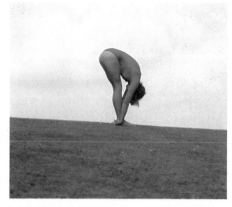

4 *Inhale*, unfolding from pelvis to upright position with legs straight and arms at sides.

5 *Exhale*, arching head and then torso backwards as slide backs of hands down legs.

6 *Inhale*, straightening to upright position by moving torso and then head. Stand with legs together. *Exhale*, repeating forward relaxation.

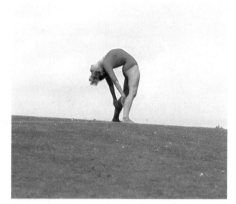

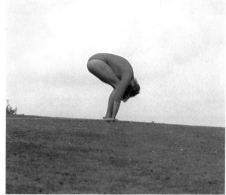

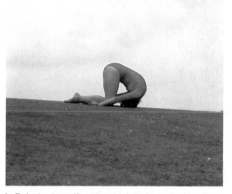

7 *Inhale*, unfolding to upright position. *Exhale*, arching backwards with legs together or astride.

8 *Inhale*, straightening to upright position. *Exhale*, relaxing forward and bending knees as head and torso start to go forward. *Inhale*, unfolding to upright position.

9 *Exhale*, kneeling down. *Inhale*, relaxing forward from waist to push over onto back of head, arms relaxed with palms uppermost. *Exhale*, sitting back on heels with body and head relaxed forward, arms relaxed, palms uppermost.

Neck and Shoulder Tension

The problem You are probably well aware that neck and shoulder tension are the first signs of impending headaches or even migraine. The basic cause is a build-up of hidden tension in the nerve centre between neck and shoulders.
The solution These movements stretch the spine and then gently twist it along its entire length, thus helping to draw out the tensions causing discomfort. When you have learned to stretch completely, you have learned to relax completely!

Breathing pattern Normal (see page 17). Hold for Complete Breaths in each maximum position.
Note Your head *always* turns in the direction of the twist. Keep your chin up and look along the appropriate shoulder. If you find it hard to balance in the Standing Twist, support yourself by standing with your back approx. 15 cms (6 ins) from a wall.

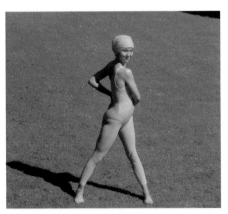

Preparation: 1 Stand with legs 60–90cm (2–3ft) apart. *Inhale* 1–5, placing left hand in small of back. *Exhale* 1–5, twisting torso to left and taking right hand to top of left thigh. *Complete Breaths.*

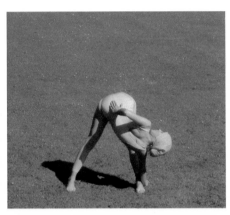

2 *Inhale* 1–5. *Exhale* 1–5, sliding right hand down outside of left leg until palm touches ground behind heel. *Complete Breaths. Inhale* 1–5, unfolding to upright position. *Exhale* 1–5. Repeat to right side.

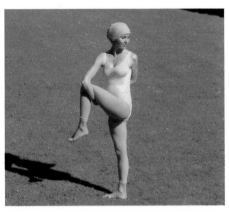

Standing Spinal Twist (Side view) Stand with legs together. *Inhale* 1–5, raising left leg and holding knee with right hand or arm under thigh. *Exhale* 1–5, twisting torso to left, hands joined behind back. *Complete Breaths.* Repeat to right.

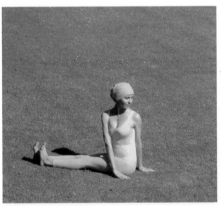

Seated Spinal Twist: 1 Sit with legs straight. *Inhale* 1–5, stretching spine upwards. *Exhale* 1–5, twisting torso to left. Note position of hands. *Complete Breaths.* Relax to starting position.

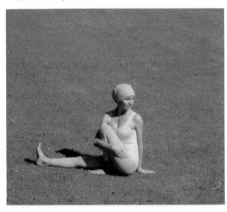

2 Draw left knee to chest as *inhale* 1–5. *Exhale* 1–5, twisting torso to left and holding left leg with right arm, left palm behind left buttock. *Complete Breaths.* Relax to starting position. Repeat, raising both knees.

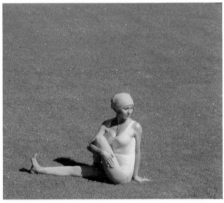

3 *Inhale* 1–5 and cross left foot over right thigh, circling left leg with right arm. *Exhale* 1–5 and repeat twist to left side. *Complete Breaths* in maximum twist position. Relax to starting position.

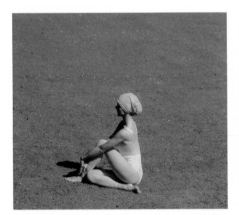

4 Bend knees, keeping feet together, and slide left hand under legs to grasp right ankle and pull foot under left thigh until knee touches back of left foot. Rest hands on left ankle. *Complete Breaths.*

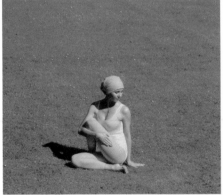

5 *Inhale* 1–5, moving left foot backwards to rest alongside right thigh. *Exhale* 1–5, twisting torso to left with right arm round raised knee and left hand pushing down to ground to stretch spine. *Complete Breaths.*

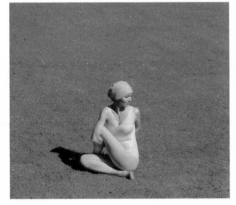

6 *Inhale* 1–5 and *exhale* 1–5, sliding right arm under raised left thigh and trying to grasp hands or wrists behind back. *Complete Breaths.* Repeat **1–6**, twisting to right side.

Headache and Migraine

The problem For many sufferers of headache and migraine the cause is the inability to let go and relax totally without feeling guilty that they should be doing something more 'constructive'.

The solution The simplicity of these very basic movements is the essence of their success. The greatest revelations can be found in stillness, and these constructive exercises should be performed very slowly with a deep awareness of the relaxation that is taking place in the neck and shoulders. This is the area which holds the tensions causing discomfort.

Breathing pattern Normal (see page 17). Only hold for Complete Breath occurs on completion of Neck and Shoulder Stretch sequence.

Note The best time to practise is when you do not have an attack.

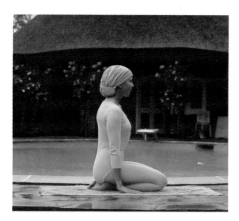
Preparation: 1 Sit on heels with hands resting gently on ground by sides and *inhale* 1–10.

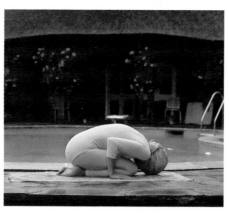
2 *Exhale* 1–10, bending forehead to ground in front of knees. Very gently rest palms of hands on ground at sides.

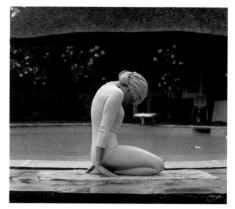
3 *Inhale* 1–10, slowly unfolding from base of spine upwards. *Exhale* and relax. Repeat **1–3** before going on to suggested programme.

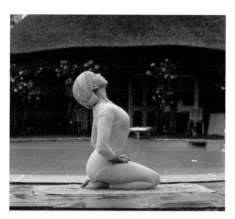
Head Roll Sitting on heels, *inhale* and *exhale*, slowly rolling head in a circle – forward, right, back, left and forward again. Feel the stretch as various parts of neck are exercised. Repeat roll 3 times in alternate directions.

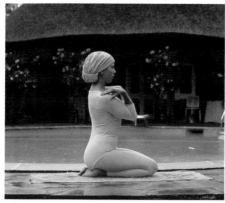
Shoulder Roll Sitting on heels, place both hands on shoulders. *Inhale*, touching elbows in front. *Exhale*, rolling arms in circular rotation up, back, and forward. Repeat 3 times in clockwise, then anticlockwise, direction.

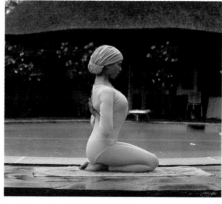
Shoulder Stretch Sitting on heels, *inhale* and *exhale*, pressing right hand up spine, palm facing outwards, using left hand to push right arm upwards. Repeat, reversing arms.

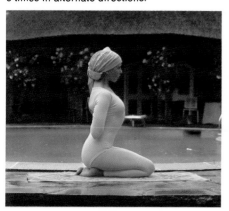
Neck and Shoulder Stretch: 1 Sitting on heels, slide right arm up spine. *Inhale* 1–10, stretching left arm up and backwards over shoulder to place left palm over right.

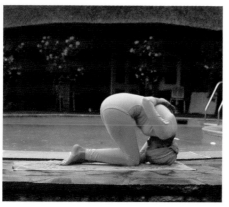
2 *Exhale* 1–10, bending forward to rest left elbow on ground in front of left knee. *Inhale* 1–10, raising hips and stretching back of neck to press crown of head on ground.

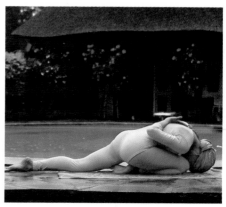
3 *Exhale* 1–10, sliding left leg straight out behind and sitting down on right foot. Rest on forehead.

Neck and Shoulder Stretch continued

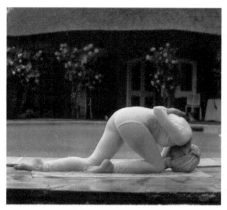

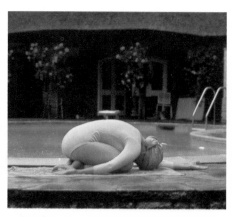

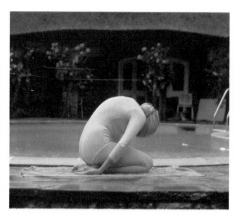

4 *Inhale* 1–10, raising hips and pressing over on crown of head to drag left leg back into seated position.

5 *Exhale* 1–10, gently massaging back of neck and head with middle finger of left hand as relax left arm forward and right arm by side, palms uppermost.

6 *Inhale* slowly, gently unfolding to upright seated position and drawing arms onto lap. *Exhale* and relax. Repeat **1–6** on other side.

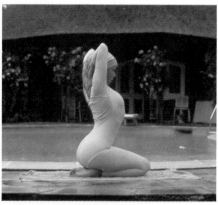

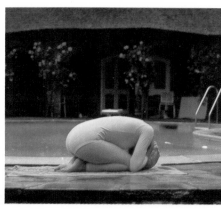

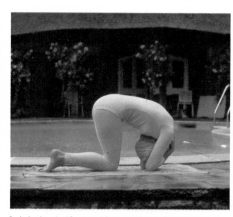

7 Still in seated position, *inhale* 1–10, raising both arms up over head and then down to rest hands on spine, left over right.

8 *Exhale* 1–10, bending forward until elbows touch floor and chin is tucked into chest.

9 *Inhale* 1–10, pushing weight forward onto elbows. Hands now slide down to cup back of neck and head rests just off ground.

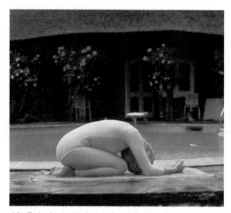

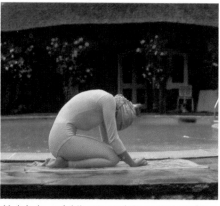

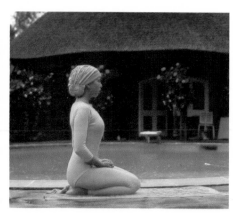

10 *Exhale* 1–10, lowering hips back onto feet as forearms relax forward, left hand still resting on top of right, palms uppermost.

11 *Inhale*, unfolding to upright seated position and dragging arms onto lap. *Exhale* as hands come to rest with palms facing upwards and tips of thumbs touching.

12 Rest for few minutes with eyes gently closed and return to natural rhythm of breathing. Repeat **1–12** on other side.

Massage can play an important part in the relief and prevention of headache and migraine.

You can perform many of these movements yourself with considerable benefit, but if you persuade a partner to help the effects are even more relaxing. The masseur finds benefit too – in laying aside his or her own problems to help another.

Try playing some restful music in the background while doing the massage. End the whole sequence by gently covering the ears with cupped hands for a few minutes. This enhances the effects of massage by eliminating external sounds.

Note All that's required for the circular pressure is a *very gentle* movement of the scalp under the thumbs, as if inscribing circles. Incidentally, the temples are the indentations at the sides of the head, level with the eyebrows.

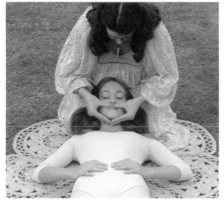

Back Traction Stand astride thighs of partner, who lies face down, arms and head to side. Hold his or her hips and pull upwards, slowly straightening your legs to take weight. Lower hips to ground. Repeat 1–6 times.

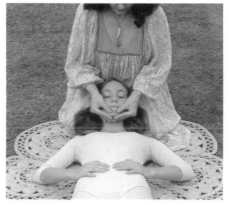

Neck Traction Sit on heels with back of partner's head on your lap, his or her knees together and raised. Place your interlaced hands under chin and pull head and neck towards you. Repeat 1–6 times.

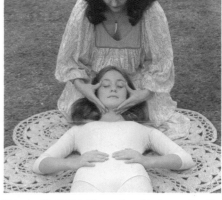

Hair and Scalp Traction Turn partner's head to left, resting chin on your left hand. Take piece of hair, close to scalp, and gently pull and rotate. Repeat all over right side. Repeat on left. Repeat cycle 1–6 times.

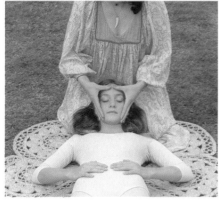

Forehead Massage Starting at partner's upper forehead, press thumbs outwards from centre to temples, ending with *gentle* circular press on temples. Repeat, working down to eyebrows. Repeat cycle 1–6 times.

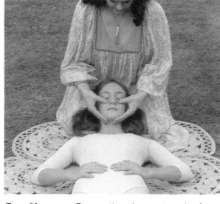

Eye Massage Press thumbs outwards from corners of partner's eye sockets in line underneath eyebrows and above eyes, ending in circular press at temples. Repeat under eyes. Repeat cycle 1–6 times.

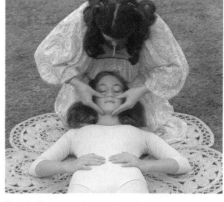

Cheek Massage Press thumbs outwards from top of partner's nose, across cheeks, to end in circular press at temples. Repeat, working down nose and curving round cheekbones and up to temples. Repeat cycle 1–6 times.

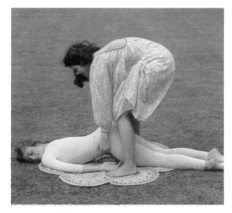

Lip Massage From under partner's nose, press thumbs out under cheeks and up to temples, ending in circular press with tips of thumbs. Repeat very gently across lips. Repeat cycle 1–6 times.

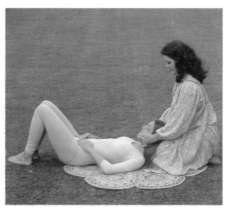

Jaw Massage Lightly pinch partner's jaw between your forefingers and thumbs at centre of chin and pull outwards along jawline to circular press at temples. Repeat 1–6 times.

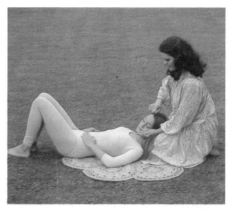

Temple Massage Place thumbs on partner's temples, resting your fingers under chin. Press thumbs *gently* in 6 clockwise and 6 anticlockwise movements, gradually making strokes lighter and lighter.

Depression and Anxiety

The problem If you haven't already read and worked on the Breathing and Relaxation section, see page 15 now. If you have, then you know how intimately your breathing habits and your thoughts are connected, and how relaxation and proper breathing calm the mind.

The solution These breathing exercises are simply an extension of the good habits you have been learning. The Complete Breath taught you how to use the full, natural power of your lungs and how to empty them thoroughly;

after a while you'll be able to draw strength and harmony from that technique by taking a few Complete Breaths as you go about your day's work. Now you are going to begin controlling and developing your breathing.

Note Go carefully with these exercises at first. Concentrate on one per session and begin by lying down to practise. Stop at once and relax in the Resting Pose (see page 15) if you feel dizzy. It's simply the unaccustomed power that all that oxygen is bringing you.

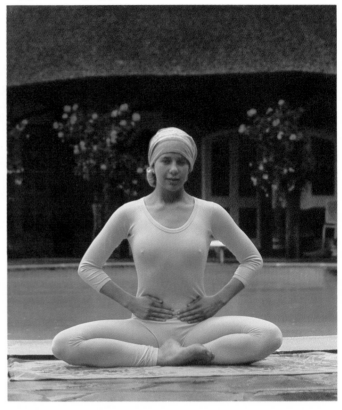

above left

Expansion Breath: 1 Sit in one of the Lotus positions (see page 37).

2 Raise both hands to chest level, placing tips of fingers together, palms downwards. *Inhale* 1–20, contracting elbows backwards as chest expands.

3 *Exhale* 1–20, bringing fingertips together again. Relax.

4 Repeat 6 times.

above

Contraction Breath: 1 Sitting in one of the Lotus positions, place hands on lower abdomen, fingertips together. *Inhale* 1–20 and *exhale* 1–20.

2 Without breathing, contract stomach 1–20 and relax 1–20.

3 *Inhale* 1–20 and *exhale* 1–20.

4 Repeat 6 times.

left

Single Nostril Breath: 1 Sit in one of the Lotus positions, both hands resting in lap.

2 Block right nostril with right thumb, other fingers extended horizontally across face.

3 *Inhale* 1–20 through left nostril. Clench fingers into fist and block nose 1–20. Relax fingers and *exhale* 1–20 through left nostril.

4 Without breathing, contract abdomen 1–20. Relax 1–20.

5 Repeat **2–3**.

6 Repeat **2–5**, blocking left nostril with left thumb.

7 Repeat on both sides 3 times.

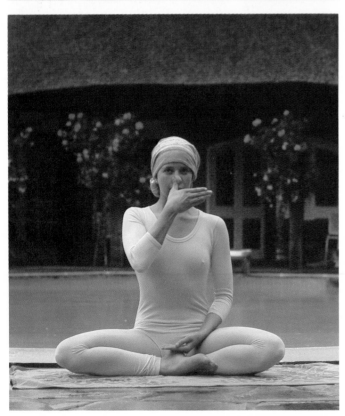

According to Indian mythology, this sequence of movements was invented as a thanksgiving to the sun, the symbol of light and energy. The gentle, warm glow I feel on completion always makes it seem quite natural to offer my own thanks too.

The effects Depression and anxiety can be lifted in just a few minutes by stretching away the tensions which build up in the solar plexus and chest. Try to practise the series 10 times a day, taking only 5–10 minutes in all.

This is an ideal series of exercises for recharging batteries, whether you are a tired housewife, a student, or business man or woman. Children also enjoy the easy, flowing movements which enhance a general sense of rhythm and natural flexibility.

Breathing pattern Normal (see page 17). No hold for Complete Breath.

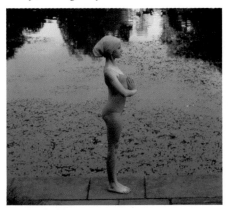

Sun Exercises: 1 Stand with legs together, arms at sides. Raise hands to solar plexus with palms facing inwards and fingertips touching. *Inhale*, palms pressing in and down as chest expands.

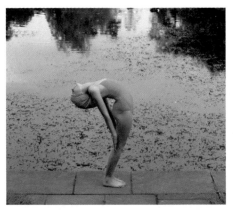

2 *Exhale*, arching torso backwards with hands pressing into backs of thighs, palms outwards, and shoulders contracted back.

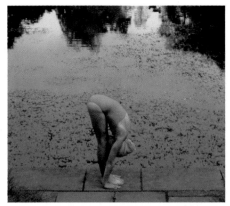

3 *Inhale* to upright position, arms at sides. *Exhale*, relaxing body downwards over straight legs, hands to ground with palms downwards.

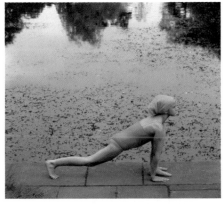

4 *Inhale*, sliding right leg back to balance on ball of foot as left knee bends. Keep head up, body in line with left thigh, and hands either side of left foot.

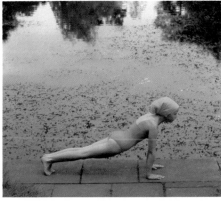

5 *Exhale*, sliding left leg back to join right. Hold position for 1–5.

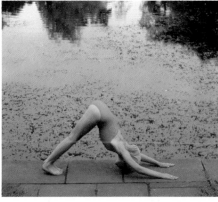

6 *Inhale*, raising hips, while arms push chin to ground and heels press downwards.

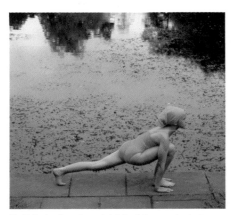

7 *Exhale*, lunging right foot forwards between arms to resume position shown in **4** (sides reversed).

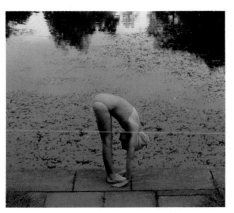

8 *Inhale*, drawing left leg in beside right and then slowly unfolding until standing with body relaxed downwards over straight legs, hands to ground with palms upwards.

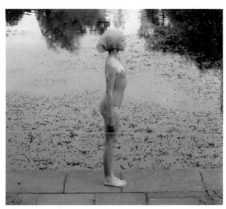

9 *Exhale*, resuming starting position, arms relaxed by sides. Rest for few minutes with eyes closed. Repeat **1–9** on other side.

Blood Pressure Problems

Establishing healthy breathing patterns is the basis of curing and preventing these problems. The natural therapy of correct breathing techniques (plus relaxation and meditation) performed for only 15 minutes every day will soon have beneficial results.

High blood pressure Use the Warrior Breath, the Heart-Beat Breath, and this variation of the Alternate Nostril Breath.

Low blood pressure Use the Heart-Beat Breath, this Alternate Nostril Breath, the Knee to Ear Pose, and the Shoulder Stand.

Note You should feel no strain while practising these breathing exercises. If you do, the best thing to do is to breathe through your mouth until the exercise becomes easier. Then, when you revert to breathing through your nostrils, lower the breath count at first.

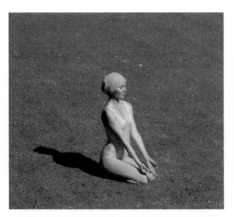

Warrior Breath: 1 Sit on heels, hands on knees in Fourth Lotus Hand Position (see page 37). *Inhale* 1–20 with 'sa' sound, as chest and ribs expand, stomach remains relaxed. *Exhale* 1–20 with 'ha' sound. Repeat 1–10 times.

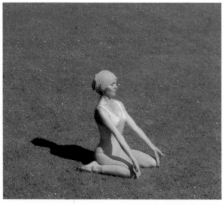

2 Move hands sideways to rest fingertips outside knees. Raise hips and move feet apart; lower hips to ground between feet. Rest hands on knees as for **1**. Repeat *Warrior Breath*, fingertips on ground on inhalation.

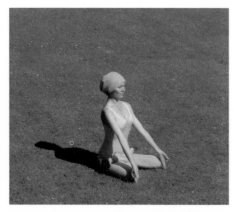

3 Fold legs into one of Lotus positions (see page 37). Repeat *Warrior Breath*, letting ribs and chest expand and relax unimpeded by extended arms.

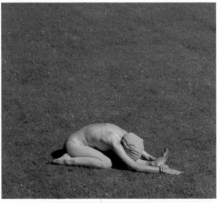

4 Sit with legs straight. Bend right leg sideways to rest foot beside hip. *Inhale* and *exhale*, holding left calf as stretch downwards, pulling torso down to lower leg. 2–3 *Warrior Breaths*. Repeat on other side.

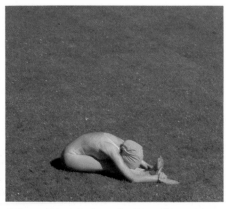

5 Repeat stretch shown in **4** but with both legs extended forward, feet flexed upwards. 2–3 *Warrior Breaths* in maximum position, relaxing from shoulders to fingertips. *Note:* chin free from chest throughout.

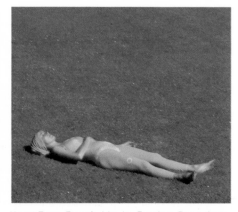

Heart-Beat Breath Lie in Resting Pose (see page 15) and place right hand over heart. Relax for few minutes, allowing heart to beat its own rhythm. 2–3 *Warrior Breaths*. Rest 15 minutes with arms at sides.

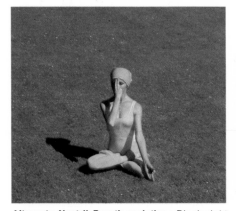

Alternate Nostril Breath variation: Block right nostril with right thumb, remaining fingers as shown. *Inhale* through left nostril 1–10. Block left nostril with curled fingers and *exhale* 1–10 through right. Reverse cycle. Repeat 1–5 times.

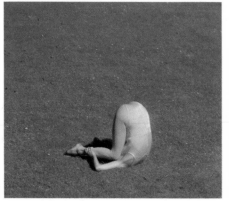

Knee to Ear Pose Lie on back, legs together. Bend knees and *inhale* 1–5. *Exhale* 1–5, pushing over into Plough (see page 47). *Inhale* and *exhale*, contracting knees to ears, and support back or legs. Relax on back. Repeat 1–5 times.

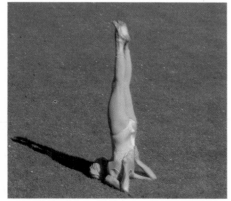

Shoulder Stand Repeat Plough, and, supporting back, contract knees to forehead before rising up to Shoulder Stand (see page 48). *Complete Breaths* through mouth until control achieved. Fold downwards and rest 15 minutes on back.

Insomnia

The source of peace and quiet is within ourselves. If we could only remember this, our minds and spirits could rest at will.
Instant relief Before getting into bed, try resting with your legs lying up the wall for 5–10 minutes. Once in bed, simply rest, applying all you've learned about relaxation and the Complete Breath (see page 15).
The solution The inverted (or upside-down) positions are often the most helpful. This is because the increased flow of blood to the head brings with it a positive sense of well-being which harmonizes all negative thoughts. The Pose of Tranquillity offers a relatively simple technique. Later you can try the Shoulder Stand (see page 48) or the Headstand (see page 49) but don't push yourself. It is much better to stay with simple routines until your body is ready.
Note Finish with relaxation and the Complete Breath.
Important See Health Precautions on page 12.

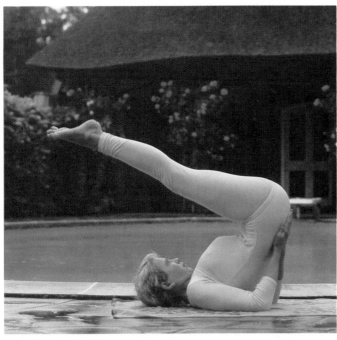

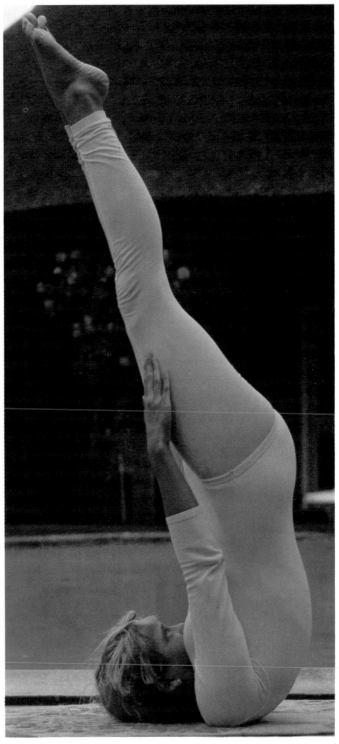

Pose of Tranquillity: 1 Lie flat on back, arms at sides. *Inhale* 1–10 and *exhale* 1–10, raising legs, with palms braced against ground to push legs back over head. Support small of back with hands. *Complete Breaths.*

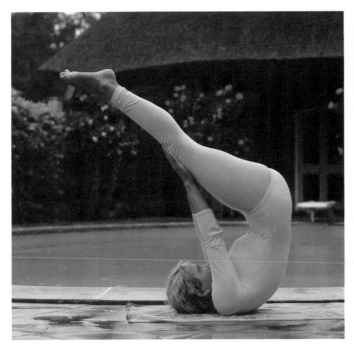

2 *Inhale* 1–10 and *exhale* 1–10, pushing torso farther off ground until body supported by shoulders, which press into ground. Place both hands, one at a time, on knees and balance. *Complete Breaths.*

3 *Inhale* 1–10 and raise torso upwards by contracting hips inwards and forwards. *Exhale* 1–10, straightening legs and resting hands on thighs. *Complete Breaths.* Slowly lower body to ground by sliding hands to hips and then rolling into Resting Pose (see page 15).

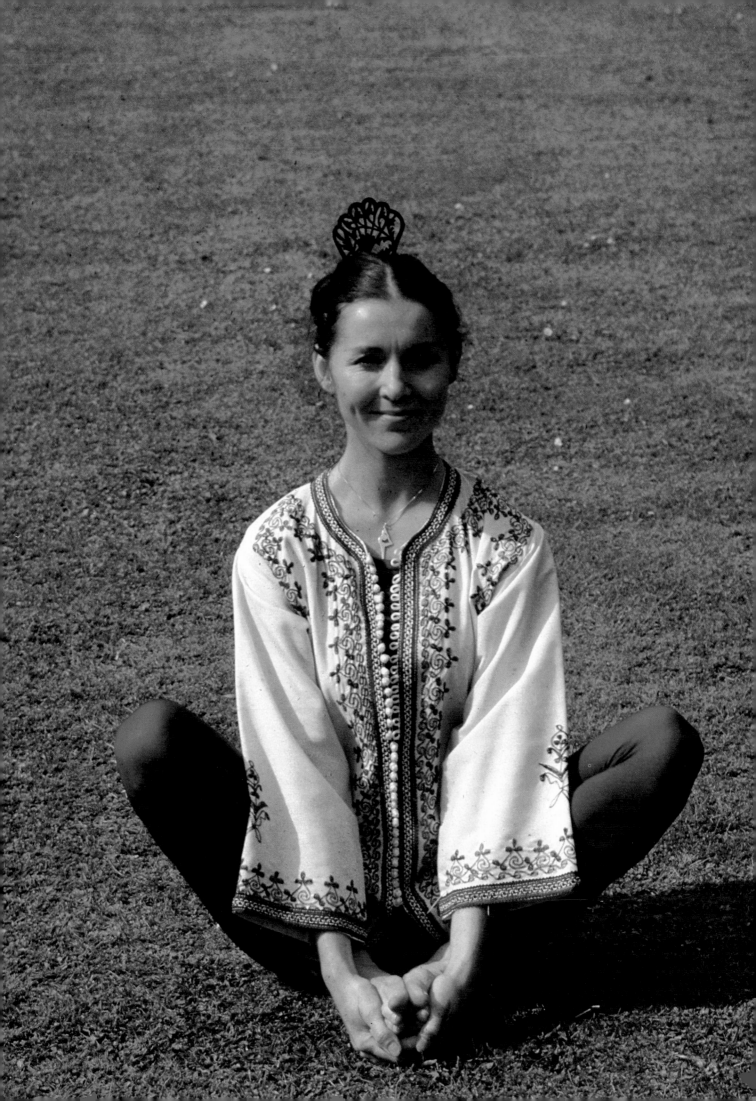

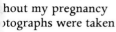

...hout my pregnancy ...and found it of great benefit. These photographs were taken ...in my sixth month.

The squat birth is quite common in India so it seemed natural to emulate this apparently effective position with exercises to be practised daily for 10-15 minutes. Expectant fathers are aware of the trials and tribulations a mother-to-be can suffer so it helps to practise the exercises together. All these exercises can be used after the birth to get your muscles back to normal.

Labour In the first stage use the Moving Squat, feet slightly apart during early contractions. Inhale and exhale slowly and deeply through mouth. See page 31 for further exercises.
Breathing pattern Normal (see page 17). No Complete Breath.
Note Moving Squat can be practised holding onto a chair.
Important Ask your doctor's permission before embarking on any exercise programme.

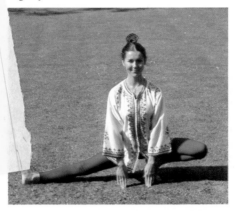

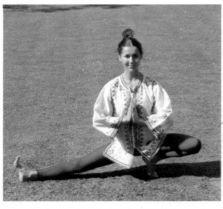

Moving Squat: 1 Stand with feet 60–90cm (2–3ft) apart, toes turned outwards. *Inhale* 1–5. *Exhale* 1–5, bending knees to squat. Fingertips touch ground in front of body. Straighten legs to rise. Repeat 6 times.

2 *Inhale* in squat and *exhale*, pushing weight over onto left foot (heel raised) and extending right leg. Push weight onto right foot and then back, maintaining continuous movement from left to right and back.

3 Repeat movement described in **2** but with palms together and pointing upwards at solar plexus.

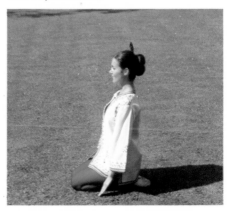

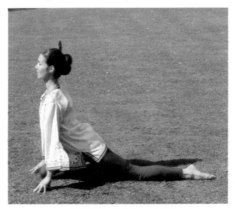

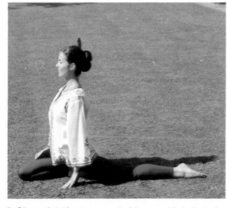

Kneeling Squat: 1 Sit on heels with arms at sides. *Inhale* 1–5, stretching spine upwards.

2 *Exhale* 1–5, raising hips and taking weight on fingertips placed alongside knees. Slide left leg back from hip joint, keeping foot relaxed.

3 Sit on right foot, arms at sides, and *inhale* 1–5. *Exhale*, raising hips and dragging left leg (knee to floor) back to position **1**. Repeat with alternate legs 6 times.

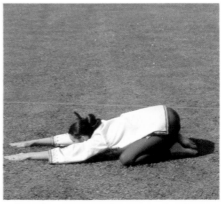

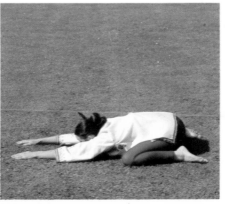

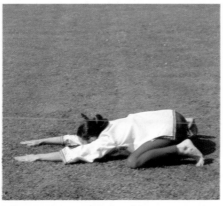

4 Open knees, arms still at sides, and *inhale* 1–5. *Exhale* 1–5, sliding arms forward along ground, palms downwards in line with shoulders. *Inhale* 1–5, returning to upright seated position, arms at sides. Repeat 6 times.

5 Raise hips and, taking weight on fingertips, move heels apart, lowering hips between feet, hands on knees. *Exhale* 1–5, sliding arms forward in line with shoulders. *Inhale* 1–5, returning to upright position. Repeat 6 times.

6 Turn toes to rest balls of feet on ground. *Exhale* 1–5 in forward stretch. *Inhale* 1–5, returning to upright position. *Exhale* and relax. Repeat 6 times.

Breathing pattern Normal. Hold for Complete Breath in Arching Squat.

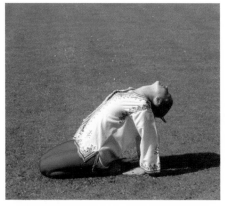

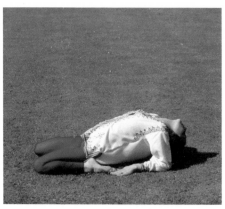

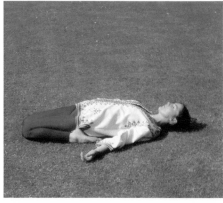

Arching Squat: 1 Sit on heels, arms at sides, and *inhale* 1–5. *Exhale* 1–5, arching head and body backwards, supporting weight on palms placed outside and behind feet. *Inhale* 1–5, straightening to upright position.

2 Raise hips to move legs apart and sit between feet. *Exhale* 1–5, arching head and body backwards. Continue backward arching movement down onto right and then left elbow. Crown of head should touch ground.

3 *Inhale* 1–5. *Exhale* 1–5, sliding head and spine flat onto ground and relaxing arms alongside body. *Complete Breath*, relaxing stomach and spine.

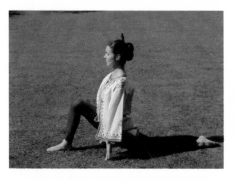

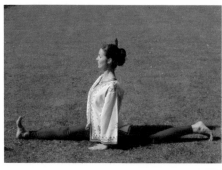

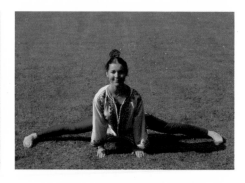

Rotation Squat: 1 Stand with legs together, arms at sides. Lunge forward with right leg, lowering left knee and fingertips to ground. *Inhale*.

2 *Exhale*, pushing hips forward and straightening right leg, keeping left leg straight. Rise by pushing weight onto hands placed either side of forward leg. Repeat 3–6 times.

3 (Side view) Position palms on left side and *inhale*, turning raised body to left, facing hands. *Exhale*, again using hands to rotate to left. Reverse semicircular movement; then repeat 1–5 times. Repeat **1–3** on other side.

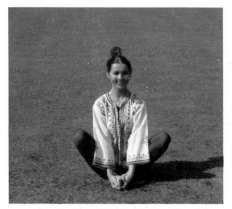

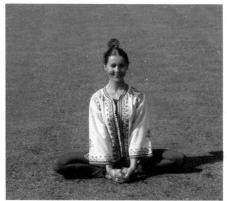

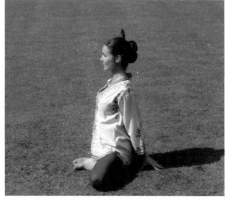

Seated Squat: 1 Sit with soles of feet touching, hands interlaced under feet. *Inhale* 1–5, contracting internal organs upwards and raising knees to shoulders.

2 *Exhale* 1–5, relaxing internal organs and hips and contracting knees down to ground while pulling feet inwards and straightening spine upwards. Repeat **1–2** 3–6 times.

3 *Inhale*, placing fingertips on ground behind body, and *exhale*, pushing weight forward onto edges of feet and contracting knees outwards.

Breathing pattern Inhale through nose and exhale through mouth, apart from panting breath, where only mouth is used. Hold for Complete Breath in Resting Squat.

Labour Resting Squat can be practised during first to third stages: **1** for first stage; **2**, between contractions, for second stage; **3** for third stage.

Toning exercises These can be practised before and after birth. But begin your after-birth exercise programme very gently with this variation of the **Contraction Breath**. *Inhale* 1–20, contracting reproductory organs, stomach and internal muscles inwards and upwards. Hold 1–20. *Exhale* 1–20, relaxing completely. Repeat 10 times a day, only returning to normal gentle exercise when it's comfortable to do so.

Note If you are unable to achieve the maximum stretch in Forward Squat, simply tilt your chin or crown of head towards ground.

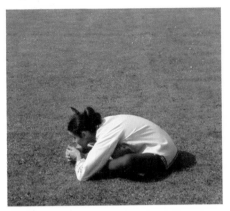

Forward Squat: 1 Sit with soles of feet touching, hands on knees. *Inhale* 1–5, sliding hands down to interlace round feet, and *exhale* 1–5, pulling spine upwards and stretching forward. Unfold upwards. Repeat 3–6 times.

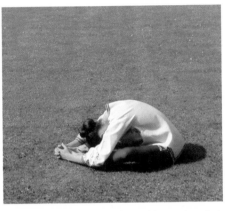

2 Repeat forward stretch, arching spine, but contract crown of head to ground between feet. Tuck chin firmly into chest and unfold to upright position, relaxing chin last. Repeat 3–6 times.

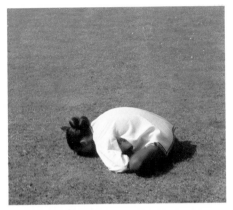

3 Placing interlaced hands round feet, draw into body. Hold big toes and *inhale* 1–5, stretching up. *Exhale* 1–5 and pull forwards, arching back, to rest chin on ground. Unfold to upright position. Repeat 3–6 times.

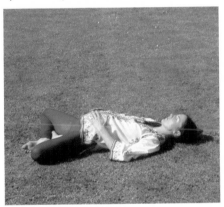

Resting Squat: 1 Lie flat on back with legs in one of first three Lotus positions (see page 37), resting hands on stomach. Gently expand on inhalation to own maximum count. Relax on exhalation. Repeat 3 times.

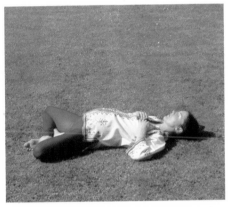

2 Rest hands on ribs or chest. Feel expansion and relaxation in 3 *Complete Breaths*.

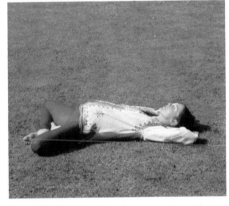

3 Rest back of neck on hands, palms uppermost. Several 'panting breaths' or *Complete Breaths*.

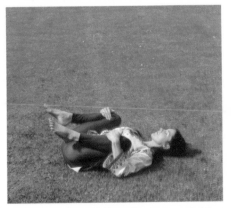

Toning Exercises: 1 Lie on back, arms at sides, palms downwards. Bracing palms on ground, raise legs at right angles to body. *Inhale* 1–5 and *exhale* 1–5, pulling knees to sides. Relax to starting position. Repeat 3–6 times.

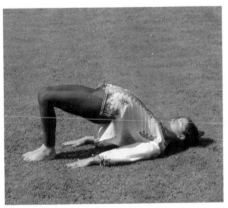

2 Bend knees and *inhale* 1–5, bracing palms on ground to raise hips and torso and contracting stomach and reproductive organs, keeping chin to chest. *Exhale* 1–5, lowering body to ground. Relax to starting position. Repeat 3–6 times.

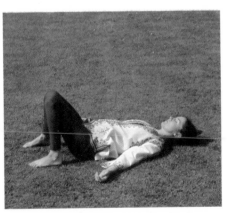

3 Relax for 5–15 minutes in Resting Pose (see page 15) or as shown, arms free from body and eyes closed while breathing to natural rhythm.

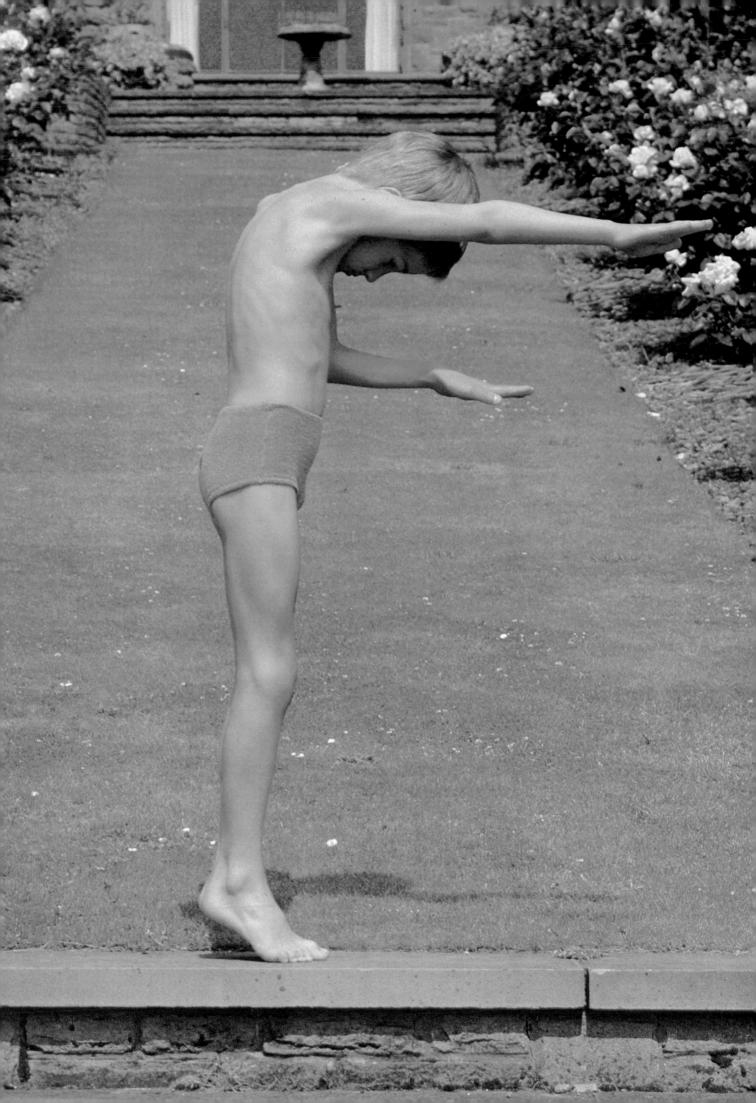

Babies and Children

Great emphasis is now put on the way we touch and care for our children. Doctors advise us more and more to show our affection not so much verbally but by loving touch, either through massage or through gentle stretching movements which help to make our children more flexible in later life. **The solution** All these exercises are designed to promote natural, healthy growth. The basic Splits is essentially very similar to the Rotation Squat given in the Pregnancy section (see page 32). It is a dynamic exercise which I have performed on my little boy since he was only a few weeks old, gradually increasing the intensity of the stretch over several months.

Once your children are old enough, encourage them to do the exercises themselves.

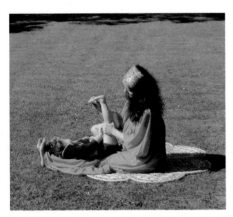

Splits: 1 Sit with legs straight. Lie baby on your legs, its head towards your feet. Straighten its right leg, holding knee and foot, and pull toes upwards and downwards to stretch tendons gently. Repeat with left leg.

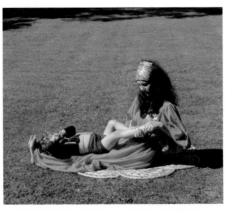

2 Take baby's right leg in both hands and pull them down leg, ending with arching stretch to ankle and toes. Lower right leg and relax. Repeat with left leg.

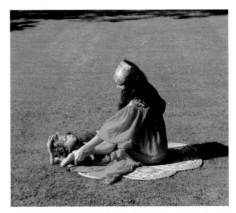

3 Grasping baby's ankles, open its legs into splits. Gently stretch right foot towards baby's ear, left foot to your right side. Bring legs together and relax. Repeat 6–12 times on alternate sides.

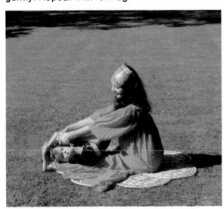

Plough: 1 Position baby and yourself as for Splits. Grasping baby's ankles, stretch both its legs over its head, trying to keep knees straight.

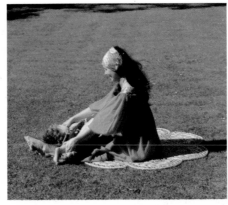

2 Continue stretch gently sideways until its feet touch ground either side of your legs. Release legs and relax.

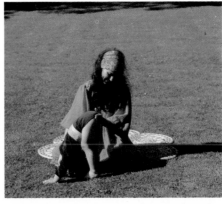

3 Sit on heels and stand baby facing sideways in front of you. Supporting its bottom, tip its body forward until head touches ground between its legs. Unfold body and relax. Repeat 6–12 times.

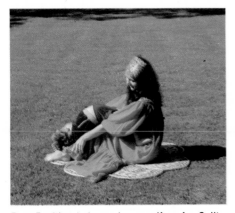

Bow Position baby and yourself as for Splits. Arch baby's body backwards by bending your knees, holding onto baby's arms. Straighten your knees and relax. Repeat 6–12 times.

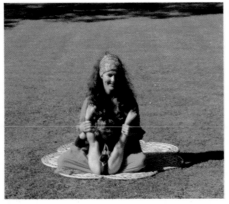

Vixen Sit on heels, knees apart, with baby between your thighs. Grasp baby's ankles and raise its legs up until either side of its head. Lower legs to ground and relax. Repeat 6–12 times.

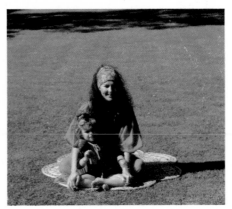

Lotus Positions as for Vixen, soles of baby's feet touching. Press baby's knees down to ground. Pull baby's right and then left leg into body, crossing left leg over right. Release legs and relax. Repeat 6–12 times.

For many children, learning the alphabet and learning to read can be difficult and tedious. This unique easy-to-follow set of movements helps by teaching the child to make the shapes of the letters with his or her own body. Letters become fun, and once the alphabet has been learned, the child can try spelling out words or even sentences.

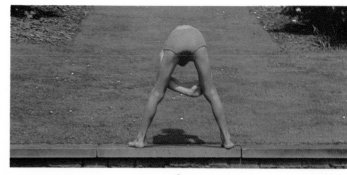

A

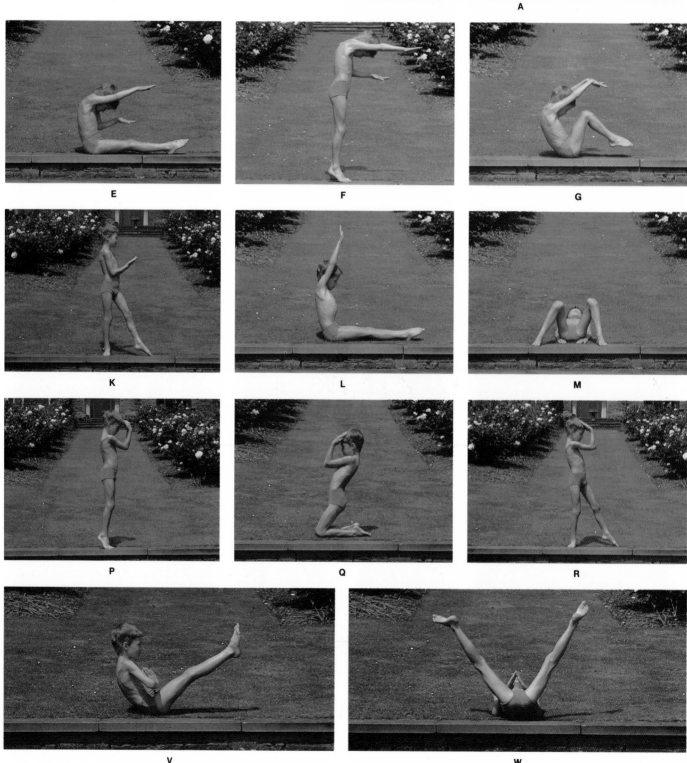

E

F

G

K

L

M

P

Q

R

V

W

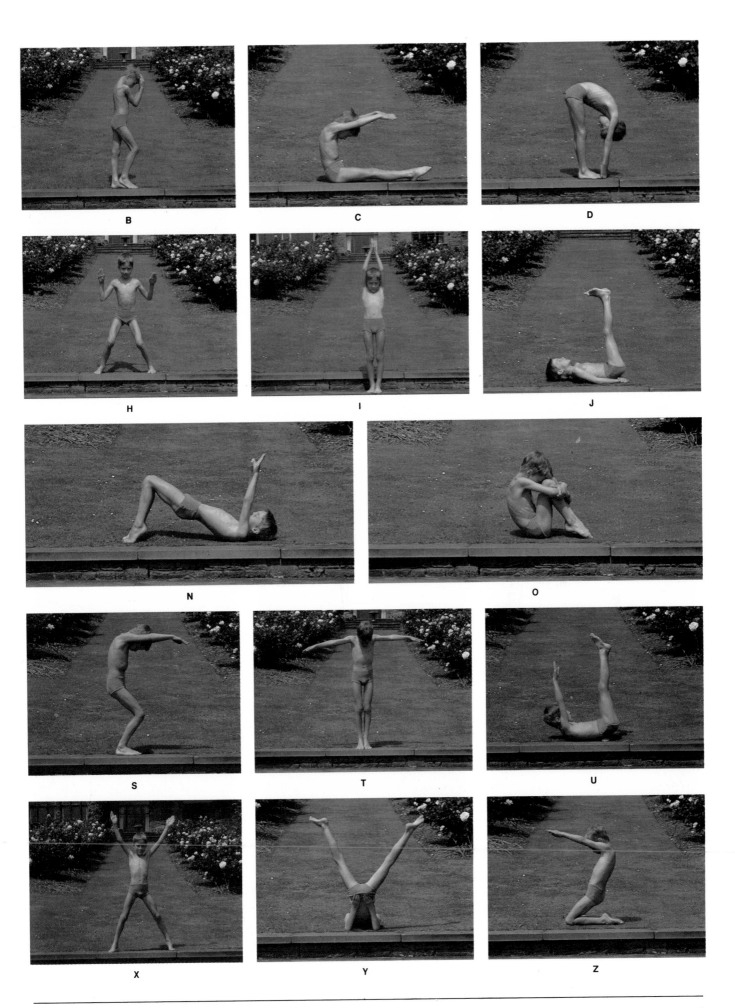

B

C

D

H

I

J

N

O

S

T

U

X

Y

Z

The Lotus exercises are among the most famous of all Yoga positions. They emulate the beautiful Indian lotus lily and carry the symbol of love: the petals of the lotus flower are represented by the legs, which, with patient practice, will open out completely.

All these Lotus exercises are good for children since they promote and maintain their natural flexibility.

Breathing pattern Normal (see page 17). No hold for Complete Breath.
Note The chin should be extended free from the chest in all the forward stretches, eyes to front unless you reach the maximum position in **5**.

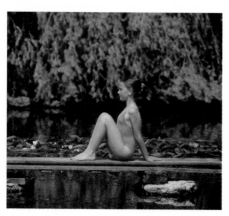

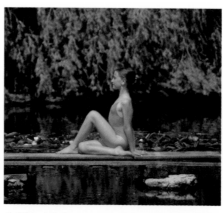

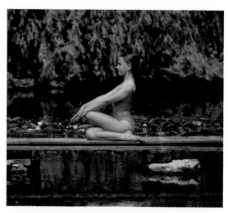

Quarter Lotus: 1 Sit with legs straight forward and body erect. *Inhale*, placing hands palms down behind back, and raise both knees.

2 Slide left hand under legs and grasp right ankle. *Exhale*, pulling right leg under raised left thigh until foot presses alongside left buttock. Return left hand to position behind back. This is the Quarter Lotus.

3 Grasp left ankle with right hand and pull foot round to right thigh. Lower knee to rest leg on right thigh. Place left hand on left knee, right on top, for Double Quarter Lotus. Lean back on hands to release legs. Repeat, reversing sides.

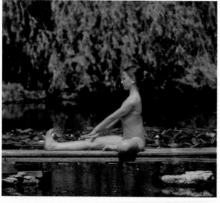

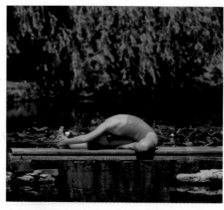

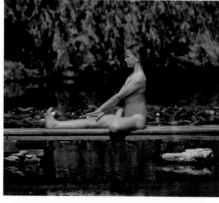

Half Lotus: 1 *Inhale*, sitting with legs straight, left hand on left knee, right on top. *Exhale* and slide hands down leg. Grasp foot, thumbs to instep, and *inhale*, sliding it up alongside right leg. *Exhale*, left hand on right on extended leg.

2 *Inhale* and *exhale*, sliding hands down extended leg. Hold maximum position, chin to lower leg or ground, and, if possible, interlace fingers round instep. *Inhale*, slowly unfolding to erect sitting position.

3 *Exhale*, lifting left foot onto lower right leg and drawing it up to thigh. *Inhale*, stretching spine upwards, and *exhale*, sliding hands and body down right leg. Unfold until upright and straighten leg. Repeat **1–3**, using right foot.

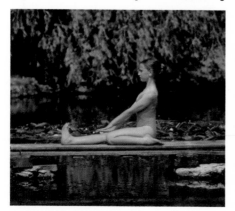

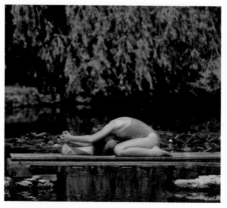

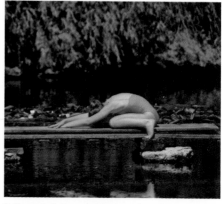

4 With legs straight forward, *inhale* and bend left knee. Holding left foot with left hand, *exhale*, pulling foot to outer side of left thigh. Lower left knee to ground. Rest left hand on right over extended right leg.

5 *Inhale* and *exhale*, sliding hands down right extended leg (toes flexed upwards). Hold maximum position, hands interlaced round instep. Slowly unfold to erect sitting position.

6 Repeat **4–5**, substituting right foot for left. Then repeat with both feet at sides. Lastly, repeat forward stretch, resting on balls of feet.

Breathing pattern Normal (see page 17), with hold for Complete Breath as each of the four positions is achieved.
Adults This series of exercises often does not come easily to the average person. Be patient with yourself if you decide to try. Several breathing and/or meditation exercises require you to sit in the Lotus position. You don't have to achieve the full pose. Choose whichever stage is most comfortable. The

important thing *is* comfort. You should be able to free your mind and body to concentrate on the exercise in hand. If at first none of them is comfortable, sit on your heels, a cushion or simply choose a straight-backed chair.

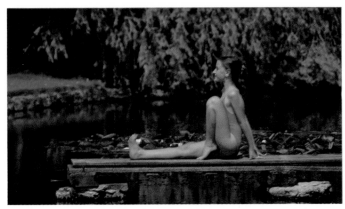

Preparation: 1 Sit with legs straight, hands braced behind back. Draw left knee into body and raise left heel, pushing weight forward onto ball of foot. Pivoting on foot, turn knee to left and groundwards, inner heel pushing forward, knee horizontal to ground.

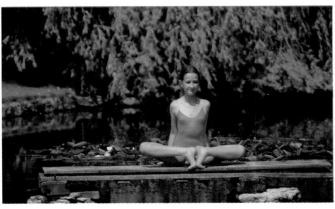

2 Slide body forward down extended right leg. Repeat, drawing right knee into body. Repeat, using both legs simultaneously.

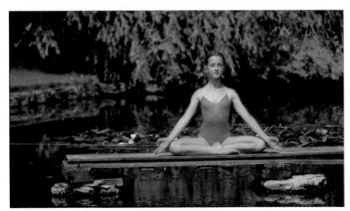

Full Lotus: 1 Extend legs straight forward, arms at sides. Pull left then right foot into body so that heels in line, knees contracted to ground and hips relaxed. Rest hands in Fourth Lotus Hand Position. *Complete Breath.*

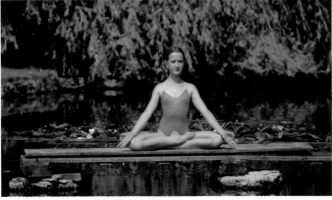

2 Grasp right foot, thumbs to instep and backs of hands facing forwards. Lift foot onto inner calf of left leg. Rest hands in Lotus position. *Complete Breath.*

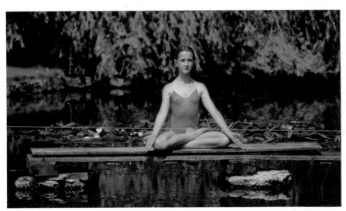

3 Grasp right foot in both hands, thumbs to instep (ankle if foot stiff), and lift onto inner thigh of left leg. Lower right knee by pressing down muscle from groin to kneecap with right palm. Rest hands in Lotus position. *Complete Breath.*

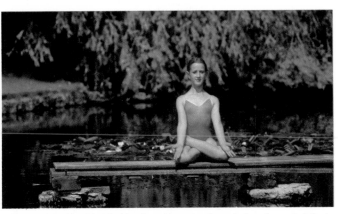

4 Brace right hand behind back and lean backwards to release left foot. Lift it over right leg onto right thigh. Rest hands in Lotus position. *Complete Breath.* Repeat, reversing sides. **Advanced Lotus:** knees tighten by flexing heels outwards.

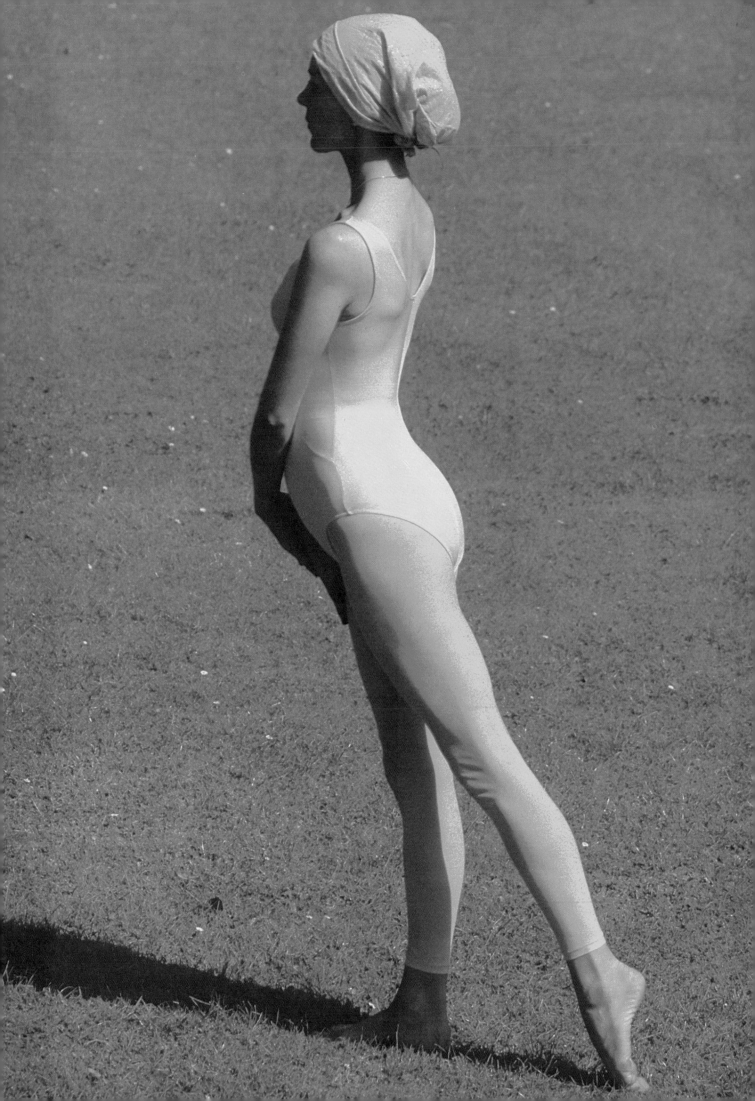

Aches, Pains and Other Ills
Sinus Congestion

The problem Phlegm, excessive mucus and sinus congestion are all indications of a system that is severely clogged. Bad headaches often accompany these conditions.

The solutions Both these breathing exercises are very helpful. Used regularly, carefully, and combined with a wholesome diet, they can cleanse the entire body system. Find out which suits you and practise the technique every day, making it the centrepiece of your session.

All the back-arching exercises, such as the Bow (see page 43) and the Cobra (see page 42), are of great benefit since they help to drain the nasal passages. Avoid the forward movements if they cause you discomfort.

Note Blow your nose gently several times before beginning the breathing exercises.

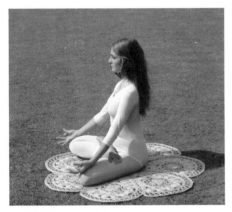

Cleansing Breath: 1 Sit in one of the Lotus positions (see page 37) on ground or in chair, with back and neck fully extended. Relax stomach and diaphragm.

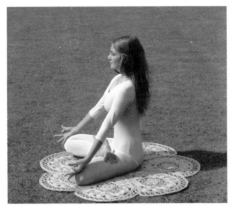

2 *Inhale. Exhale* much faster than inhalation, strongly contracting abdomen and diaphragm like pair of bellows.

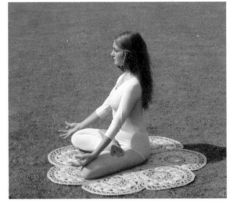

3 *Inhale* as soon as breath expelled, relaxing abdomen and diaphragm. Repeat inhalation and exhalation in quick succession 10–20 times. Follow with slow breath in and out. Relax for few minutes before next exercise.

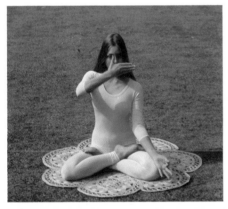

Alternate Nostril Breath: 1 Sitting in one of Lotus positions, press right thumb gently along right side of nose into inside corner of *eye socket*, other fingers extended horizontally across face. *Inhale* through left nostril 1–10.

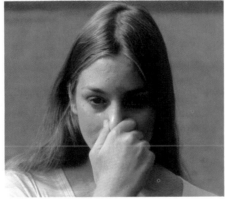

2 Block both nostrils by clenching fingers into fist. Hold breath 1–10.

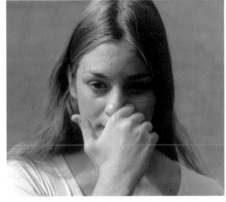

3 Release thumb, continuing to press other fingers against left nostril. *Exhale* 1–10 through right nostril. Repeat **1–3** 5 times.

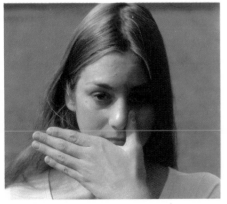

4 Press left thumb along left side of nose into inside corner of eye socket, other fingers extended across face. *Inhale* 1–10 through right nostril.

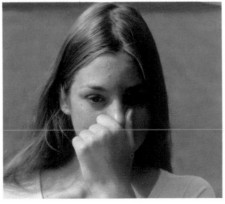

5 Block both nostrils by clenching fingers into fist. Hold breath 1–10.

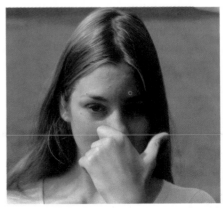

6 Release thumb, continuing to press other fingers against right nostril. *Exhale* 1–10 through left nostril. Repeat **4–6** 5 times.

Sore Throats

All these exercises can be practised when you have a sore throat or a bad cold and will bring almost immediate relief. The series of gentle massage exercises are designed to stimulate the circulation of blood to the throat, bringing relief to the affected areas.

Note Go carefully with the massage. All that's required is a very gentle pressure under your fingers or thumbs as if inscribing circles.

Throat Relaxation: 1 Gently swallow to relax throat.

2 Relax tongue, making sure it does not touch roof of mouth.

3 *Inhale* 1–5 through nose if possible, feeling cool air relax back of throat, chest, and lungs.

4 *Exhale* 1–5, feeling warm air soothing throat and expelling impurities within.

5 Repeat 1–6 times.

Lion: 1 Sit on heels or in one of the Lotus positions (see page 37), palms resting on knees.

2 *Inhale* strongly, through nostrils if possible.

3 *Exhale* with a roar, tongue fully extended out of mouth.

4 Repeat 5–10 times.

Lion variation: 1 Choose one of the Lotus positions (see page 37).

2 Rocking slightly back and then forwards, push up onto knees.

3 Walk hands forwards under shoulders. *Inhale* through nostrils 1–10, pushing hips forward to ground, head arched back, elbows slightly bent and pulled into waist.

4 *Exhale* with a roar, tongue extended.

5 Repeat 5 times.

Sun: 1 Choose one of the Lotus positions (see page 37).

2 Raise and cross arms, placing hands on opposite shoulders with elbows up in front of body. *Inhale* 1–10, arching head and neck backwards and raising elbows up over head.

3 Hold 1–10.

4 *Exhale* 1–10, returning to erect Lotus position with backs of hands resting on knees, fingers relaxed. Repeat 1–5 times.

Sun variation: 1 Sit on heels, knees and feet together.

2 Press palms together at solar plexus, wrists following natural line of ribcage.

3 Repeat Sun breathing exercise as above.

Leaf: 1 Extend tongue out of mouth and curl it into tube.

2 Gently *inhale* 1–10 through tongue.

3 Relax and retract tongue, swallow, and lock chin to chest for 1–10 counts. Release chin. *Exhale* 1–10.

4 Repeat 5–10 times, feeling cool air soothe throat.

Leaf variation: 1 Lie on stomach with legs together and arms at sides.

2 Arch body up into Cobra (see page 42).

3 Repeat Leaf breathing exercise as above.

Cobra variation A: 1 Lie on stomach with forehead to ground and legs 60–90cm (2–3ft) apart.

2 *Inhale* 1–15, arching head, then torso up and back into Cobra (see page 42).

3 Hold arched position with help of hands, and *exhale* 1–15 through mouth with tongue flat and fully extended to chin.

4 Relax torso and then chin and forehead to ground.

5 Repeat 5 times.

Cobra variation B: 1 Repeat as for variation A, but with legs together. Shoulders should be contracted back, chest expanded, and elbows slightly bent into waist in maximum position for both variations.

2 Repeat 5 times.

3 Relax with arms alongside body, palms uppermost, elbows bent outwards, head turned to side, and eyes resting.

Throat Massage: 1 Turn head slightly to right side, making the muscle joining ear to top of breast bone stand out. Using pad of one thumb, gently apply pressure to inner part of muscle in a downward direction. Turn head to left side and repeat action.

2 Stroke and gently massage trachea from top (under centre of chin) to bottom (at base of throat). Repeat several times.

3 Tap gently with 'flats' of fingers on each side of and on trachea.

4 Massage below chin with fingers of both hands, working down outside of throat.

Chilblains

The problem Poor circulation in the hands and feet is the basic cause of this irritating winter condition which afflicts people of any age.

The solution These exercises are designed to help improve circulation. They are best practised in the summer before the discomfort of chilblains begins to limit your movements. Try also the Moving Squat (see page 29) and the First Standing Pose (page 44).

Breathing pattern I've given the most minimal guidance for this sequence because it is much more important to *feel* the various stretches as they occur. Hold for Complete Breath in **9**. **Note** If you find balancing difficult in **7–9**, try leaning against a wall.

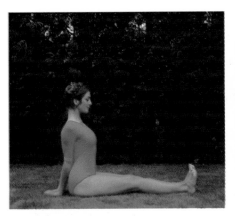

Lotus Foot and Ankle Stretch: 1 Sit with legs straight. Place hands, palms downward, immediately behind back.

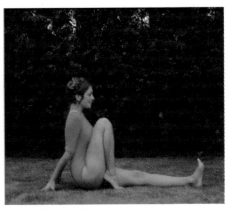

2 With heel raised, draw right foot up to body, bracing erect body against arms.

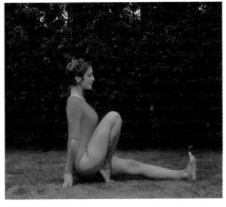

3 Raise both hips, taking weight on fingertips. Right knee should be directly above right ankle, heel still raised.

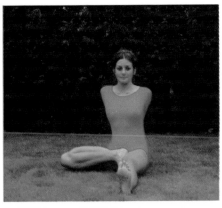

4 Pivot ball of right foot outwards, contracting right knee to side, while pushing body forward with shoulders contracted backwards and hands braced close together behind back. Sit down behind raised heel.

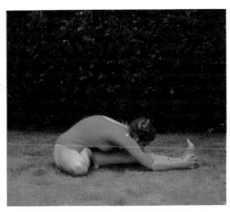

5 *Inhale* and *exhale*, stretching head and body forwards and down extended left leg to interlace fingers under instep or round ankle. Keep chin away from chest.

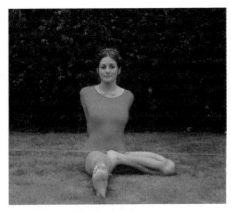

6 Repeat **1–5**, using left leg.

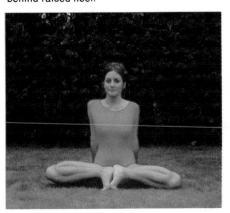

7 Repeat sequence, drawing both feet simultaneously into body, relaxing hips and contracting knees to ground. Sit erect with heels raised and balls of feet touching, hands braced behind back.

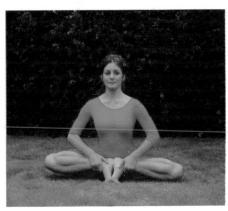

8 Grasp raised ankles and push hips down to ground behind feet.

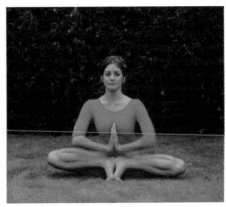

9 Balance in maximum stretch with palms together at solar plexus (in First Lotus Hand Position). *Complete Breath.*

Chest Complaints

The problem Rounded shoulders and stooping stance can affect not only your whole outlook on life but indeed the very health of your body. Asthma and bronchitis are certainly associated with bad posture, and premature ageing (as well as many internal disorders) can be caused by the compression of internal organs. Blood ceases to flow normally and no longer performs its tasks of renewing ageing cells and bearing away toxins so effectively.

The solution All these exercises are excellent correctives. You can also help yourself by walking tall, keeping your shoulders back and down. Don't tense them. Drawing your weight up off the hips tones up your body and your mind.
Breathing pattern Normal (see page 17), holding maximum stretches for Complete Breath.
Note All three exercises can be practised standing up. Finish by relaxing the lumbar region (see page 44, Instant relief).

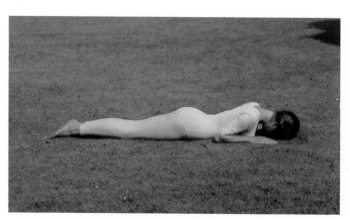

Cobra: 1 Lie on stomach, forehead to ground, with ankles, knees and hips contracted. Place hands either side of head so that parallel lines could be drawn from wrists to elbows. Fingers should be fully extended.

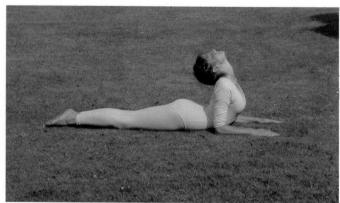

2 *Inhale* 1–10, arching head, then shoulders, chest and ribs backwards. Eyes guide head movement, up and back, while forearms remain flat on ground. *Exhale* 1–10. *Complete Breath*. Relax to ground.

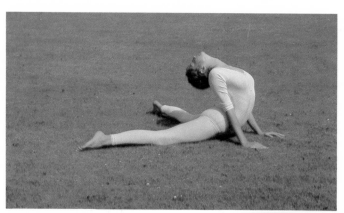

3 Slide hands back, raising elbows above wrists, and repeat **2**. Repeat with legs 60–90cm (2–3ft) apart. Keep shoulders contracted back and elbows slightly bent into waist.

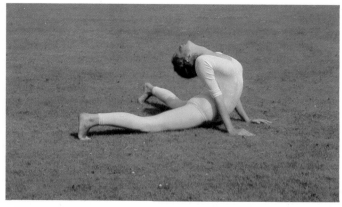

4 With hands positioned as for **3** and legs apart, rise onto balls of feet and repeat Cobra arch, keeping hips to ground. *Complete Breath*. Relax ribs, chest, chin, forehead and toes to ground.

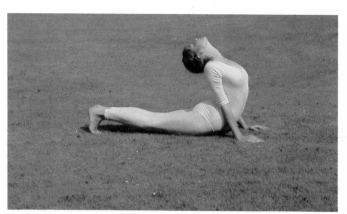

5 Repeat Cobra arch with legs together and using balls of feet. Raise thighs off ground if possible. *Complete Breath* in maximum position. Relax to ground.

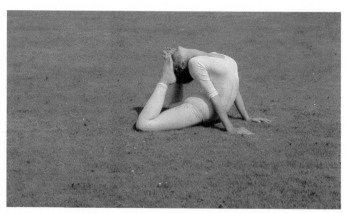

6 With legs together or apart, arch into Full Cobra, raising feet to head or shoulders. *Complete Breath* in maximum position and then relax to ground with head to one side, shoulders relaxed, arms by sides with elbows slightly bent and palms uppermost.

Breathing pattern Normal (see page 17). No holds for Complete Breath.
Note If 1 proves too difficult, try holding the foot with just one hand.

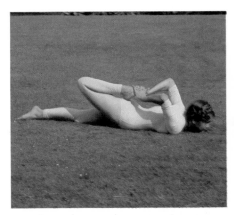

Bow: 1 Lie on stomach, resting chin on ground. Bend right leg and interlace fingers below toes, thumbs to instep. *Inhale* 1–5 and *exhale* 1–5, pulling right foot into small of back. Repeat with left foot.

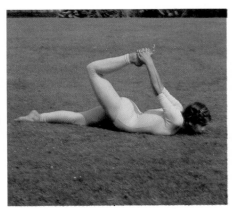

2 Bend right leg and interlace fingers and thumbs below toes. *Inhale* 1–5, pushing right foot upwards and forwards until arms are fully extended. *Exhale* 1–5, lowering leg to ground. Repeat with left foot.

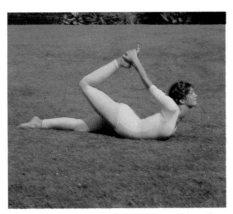

3 Repeat **2**, arching head and shoulders back on inhalation. Repeat **1–2**, using both legs simultaneously and starting with legs apart. Repeat with legs together.

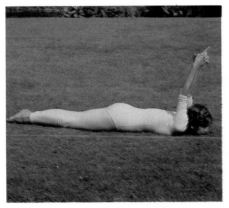

Jack Knife: 1 Lie on stomach with chin on ground and interlace fingers behind back, forefingers extended. *Inhale* 1–10, raising arms up and forwards. *Exhale* 1–10, lowering arms to sides. Relax, head to side.

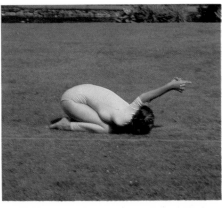

2 Sit on heels, arms at sides. Interlace fingers behind back, forefingers extended. *Inhale* 1–10, raising arms and stretching body and arms forwards to rest chin on ground. *Exhale* 1–10, lowering arms. Relax.

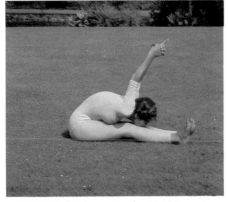

3 Sitting with legs straight, repeat **2**, flexing feet inwards on forward stretch and resting chin on knees. Sitting with straight legs apart, repeat **2**, bringing chin down to ground and again flexing feet upwards.

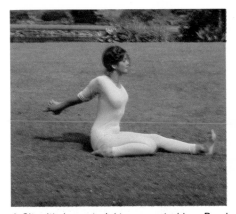

4 Sit with legs straight, arms at sides. Bend right leg gently sideways and back until foot rests beside right hip. Interlace fingers behind back, forefingers fully extended.

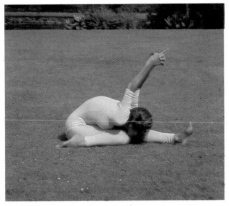

5 *Inhale* 1–10, stretching forwards, until arms over head and chin touches left leg or ground. *Exhale* 1–10 on maximum stretch and relax upwards. Repeat **4–5**, reversing sides. Repeat with both legs bent, sitting between heels.

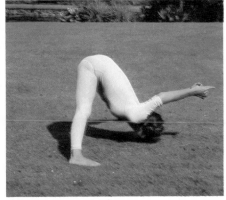

6 Standing with legs 60–90cm (2–3ft) apart, interlace fingers behind back, forefingers extended, and *inhale* 1–10. *Exhale* 1–10, stretching forward and down between legs. Unfold upwards. Repeat with legs together.

Back Ache

The problem Bad posture causes back complaints, especially slipped disc and lumbago. (See page 42 for other effects.)
Instant relief Severe back ache often makes exercise difficult. This simple relaxation technique can bring great relief. Lie on your stomach, head and arms to side, with elbows slightly bent and palms uppermost. *Inhale* 1–20, expanding stomach and relaxing lumbar region, hold 1–20 and *exhale* 1–20. Relax. Repeat for 2–3 minutes.
The solutions All these exercises will strengthen the muscles around your vertebrae, thus preventing slipped discs and helping to cure back ache. Hanging by your arms from a rail or doorway for just a few minutes every day is also an excellent way of stretching out hidden spinal tensions.
Breathing pattern Normal (see page 17), holding for Complete Breath in First Standing Pose.
Note If balance is difficult, 1–3 of the First Standing Pose can be practised holding onto a chair (see page 60).

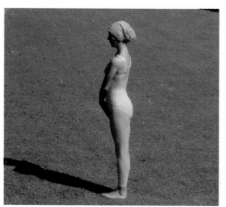

First Standing Pose: 1 Standing erect with legs together, place right palm on right thigh, left palm on top of it. *Inhale* 1–10, stretching spine upwards.

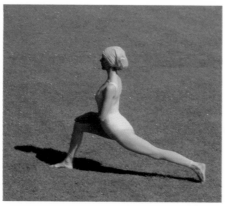

2 *Exhale* 1–10, lunging left leg backwards and keeping weight evenly distributed between both feet, hands still resting on right thigh. Right leg is now bent and left leg balances on ball of foot.

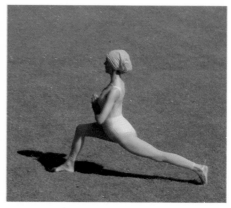

3 Return to natural rate of breathing, and, keeping body square and at same height, place palms together (thumbs crossed) at solar plexus. Raise and lower right heel 3–6 times.

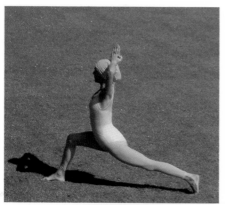

4 Still balancing with forward leg at right angles to body, *inhale* and *exhale*, raising wrists to rest on crown of head, palms together. *Complete Breath.*

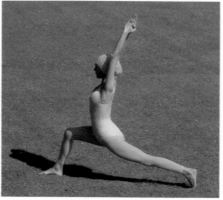

5 *Inhale* and *exhale*, arms fully extended over head, palms together. *Complete Breath.*

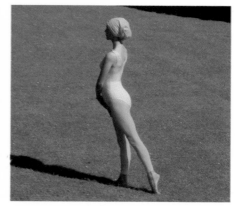

6 Lower arms to right thigh as for **2**. Lunge down, up and over onto left toes, dragging left leg back into starting position. Repeat on the other side.

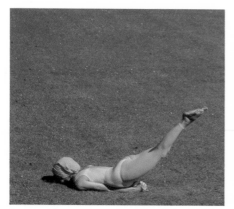

Locust: Lie face down, chin on ground, fingers interlaced and thumbs extended, or palms flat. Contract hips together and down. *Inhale* and *exhale*, raising legs and hips. Hold. Lower legs and relax, arms to side. Repeat 3 times.

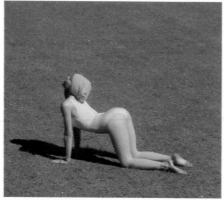

Cat Kneel with arms and legs at right angles to body. *Inhale* 1–10, hollowing back and arching head up and backwards. *Exhale* 1–10, contracting hips and head and arching back. Keep arms fully extended throughout. Repeat 3 times.

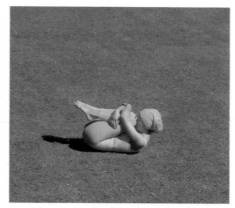

Hug Lie flat on back and draw knees up to chest. Clasping legs, gently rock from side to side while pressing lumbar region to ground. *Inhale* and *exhale*, raising forehead and then chin to touch knees; repeat 6 times.

Constipation

The problem Incorrect diet and lack of exercise play an important part. What's not commonly recognized is that stress, or depression, can affect the way we practise a harmonious diet and exercise programme.

The solutions Practise one of these exercises 10 times a day and try to take a daily walk to get fresh air too. Colitis, which is the result of severe constipation, has been cured by several of my students. The exercise programme is the same with the addition of the Headstand (see page 49), the Shoulder Stand (see page 48), and the Sleep Pose.

Sleep Pose For those who find the exercises below impossible, this is a useful alternative. Sit between feet and lie back with arms overhead. Fold hands under head and take several **Bellows Breaths**: *inhale*, relaxing stomach, and *exhale*, contracting stomach and reproductory organs deeply. Repeat for as long as is comfortable. If you have difficulty with this position, lie on back with knees raised and feet apart.

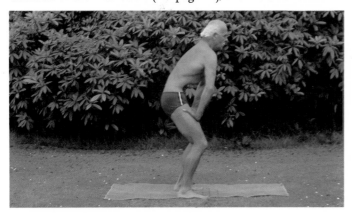

Abdominal Uplift Stand with legs 60–90cm (2–3ft) apart, arms at sides. Bending knees, lean forward and press palms down on thighs, fingers inwards. *Inhale* 1–10 and *exhale* 1–10. Contract abdominal and reproductive muscles, holding for 5–10 and then relax. *Inhale* 1–10 and *exhale* 1–10. Repeat 1–10 times.

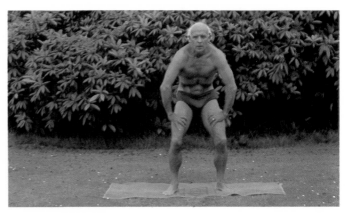

Abdominal Muscle Waving Preparing as for Uplift, *inhale* 1–10 and *exhale* 1–10. Contract abdominal area to spine. Relax side muscles and push central abdominal muscle forward. Hold 1–10. Relax. *Inhale* 1–10 and *exhale* 1–10. Repeat 1–10 times.

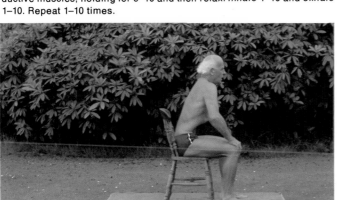

1 Repeat Abdominal Uplift or Waving 1–10 times, seated on chair with feet apart and hands pressing down on thighs or knees.

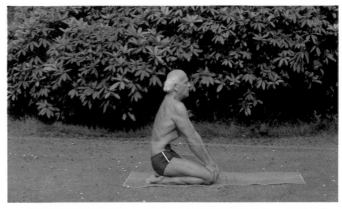

2 Repeat Abdominal Uplift or Waving 1–10 times, sitting on heels with toes overlapped or between feet, pressing hands down on thighs or knees.

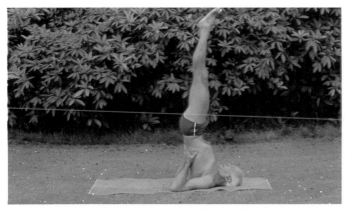

3 Repeat Abdominal Uplift or Waving 1–10 times in Plough (see page 47) or Shoulder Stand (see page 48), hands supporting back throughout.

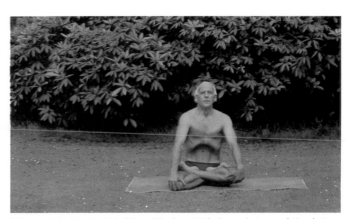

4 Repeat Abdominal Uplift or Waving 1–10 times in one of the Lotus positions (see page 37), hands pressing down on thighs or knees.

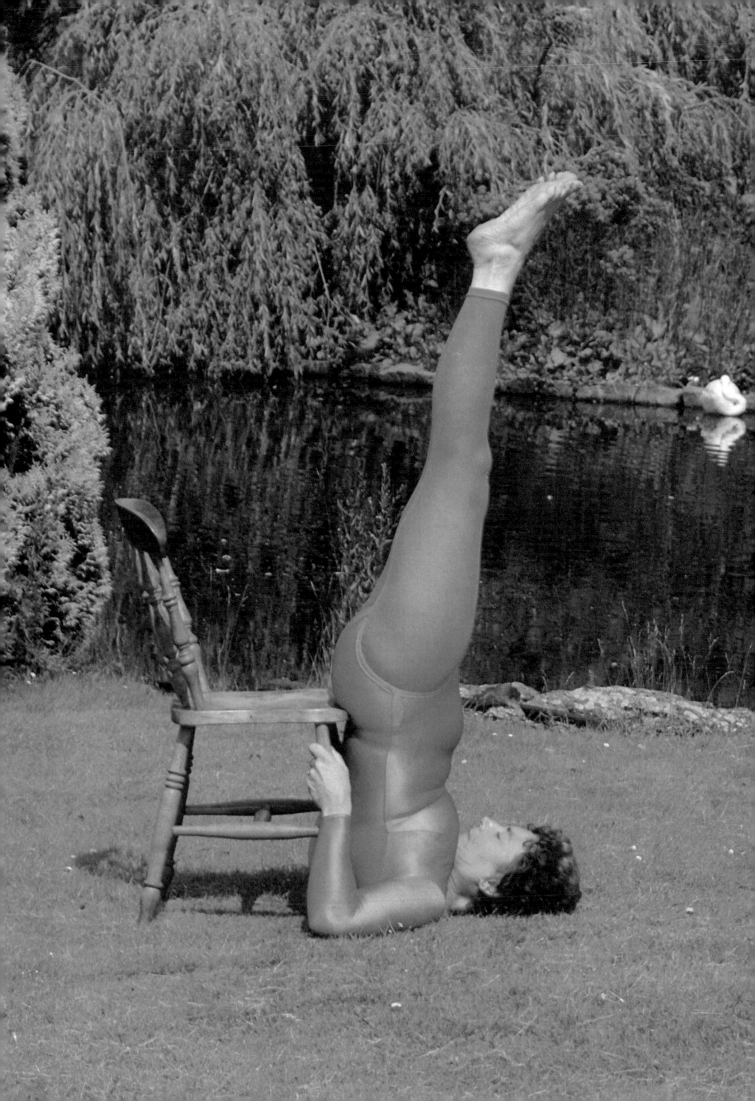

Weight Control

The problem When you're tired and overworked (or bored and underoccupied), it is all too easy to try regaining lost energy through unnecessary eating. And on a more physiological level the action of the thyroid gland is closely related to weight control and general youthfulness.

The solutions These classical Yoga poses act as a physical and mental tonic. The flexibility of the spinal column, essential to all good health, is restored and protected, and under compression in the inverted (or upside down) poses the thyroid benefits from an increased blood flow.

Side benefits These exercises help prevent ageing by increasing the blood supply to the face. Constipation and menstruation problems are also helped.

Breathing pattern Normal (see page 17).

Note Try to curb your appetite by having a warm, relaxed bath and then practising for 10–15 minutes before a meal. That way you eat more slowly and sensibly.

Important See Health Precautions on page 12.

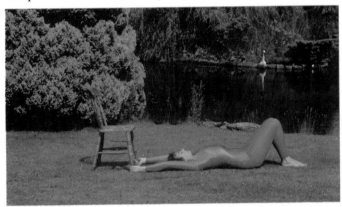

Plough: 1 Place chair within comfortable reach as shown. Lie on back with straight legs together, arms at sides. *Inhale* 1–5, taking arms back over head to check chair and raising knees while keeping feet together.

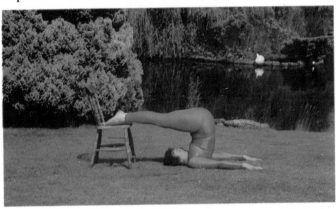

2 *Exhale* 1–5 and, bracing arms (palms downwards) by sides, raise feet to straighten legs and then lift hips and torso up, continuing movement of legs until they rest on chair seat.

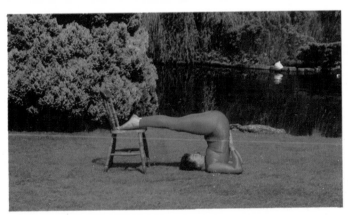

3 *Inhale* 1–5 and *exhale* 1–5, supporting back with palms of hands. Torso should be in vertical line to ground, if possible.

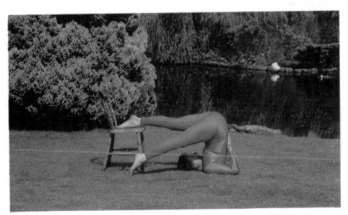

4 *Inhale* 1–5 and *exhale* 1–5, lowering right foot to ground beside chair while still supporting back. *Inhale* 1–5, returning foot to chair seat.

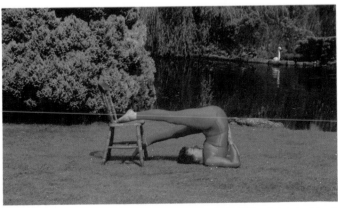

5 *Exhale* 1–5, lowering left foot to ground. *Inhale* 1–5, raising foot back onto seat.

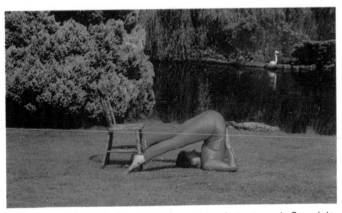

6 *Exhale* 1–5, lowering both feet simultaneously to ground. *Complete Breaths*. Raise both feet simultaneously to chair. Pressing palms to ground, slowly lower body to starting position.

Breathing pattern Normal (see page 17).

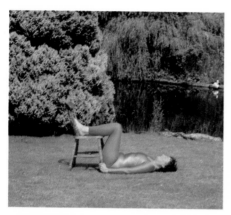

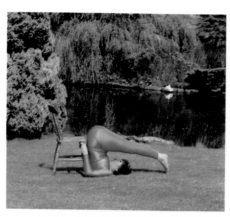

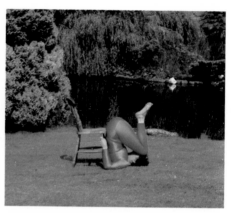

Shoulder Stand: 1 Lie on back, arms at sides, with hips between front chair legs, and feet and lower legs resting on seat. Grasp front chair legs and *inhale* 1–5.

2 *Exhale* 1–5, straightening legs over head and then (pulling chair against back for support and slowly moving hands up chair legs) gently lower legs until toes touch ground behind head.

3 *Inhale* and *exhale*, bending knees onto forehead. Feet should be directly in line with and above knees, with ankles, knees and hips locked together.

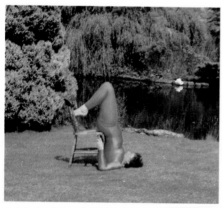

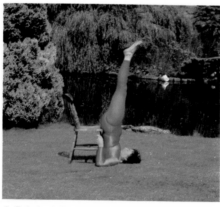

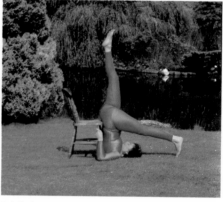

4 *Inhale* 1–5, arching contracted hips backwards and raising knees until torso and upper legs form vertical line with weight on shoulders. Feet should hang towards chair seat and chin tuck into chest.

5 *Exhale* 1–5, raising relaxed feet until legs fully extend into Shoulder Stand. *Complete Breaths*.

6 *Inhale* 1–5 and *exhale* 1–5, lowering straight right leg until toes touch ground behind head. *Inhale* 1–5, raising right leg back to Shoulder Stand. *Exhale* 1–5, repeating action with left leg. *Exhale* in Shoulder Stand.

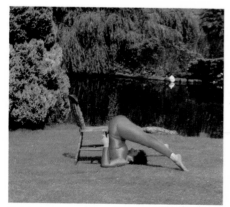

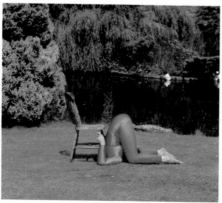

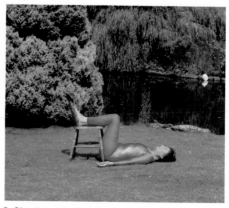

7 *Inhale* 1–5 and *exhale* 1–5, lowering both feet simultaneously to ground, feet apart in line with shoulders.

8 *Inhale* 1–5 and *exhale* 1–5, bending knees inwards to touch ground in front of shoulders. *Complete Breath. Inhale*, straightening legs, and *exhale*, clasping backs of knees to draw legs inwards as before.

9 Slowly push chair back to original position as raise knees and gently lower legs back to starting position. Rest with arms free from body, palms uppermost, and return to natural breathing rhythm.

This series of head-to-toe **Yogatone Exercises** should be coupled with the weight control formula described on pages 47–48 and can be used by people of all ages. If you are unable to do the Tree or Stork Lotus, simply perform the Complete Stork Lotus sequence with both legs together.
Side benefits The balanced positions help improve general posture and carriage. Regular practice also benefits cramp and poor circulation.

Breathing pattern Normal (see page 17).
Note If you have difficulty in keeping your balance, ask someone to hold you for support or try using a wall.

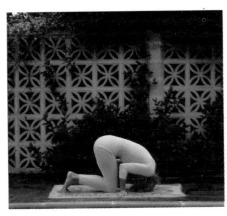

Headstand: 1 Sit on heels, arms at sides, and *inhale. Exhale*, bending head and torso forward placing palms at right angles to and in front of knees. Raise hips and, resting on balls of feet, continue forwards until crown touches ground.

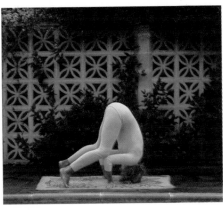

2 Taking body weight onto hands, *inhale* and begin straightening legs until knees are raised to rest on elbows. *Exhale*, bending knees again and taking feet up to thighs.

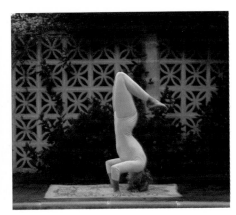

3 Draw knees into armpits. *Inhale*, arching back and raising knees, keeping feet to buttocks, until knees are directly above head.

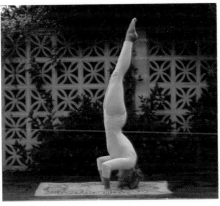

4 *Exhale*, extending legs upwards over head into Headstand. Relax feet and legs to allow blood to flow freely. *Complete Breaths*.

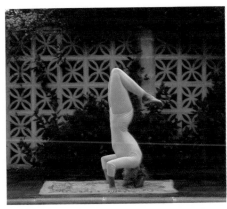

5 *Inhale* and *exhale*, bending knees to bring feet down to buttocks.

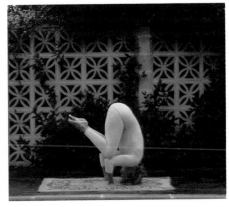

6 *Inhale* and *exhale*, continuing downward folding movement by bringing knees down to rest on upper arms.

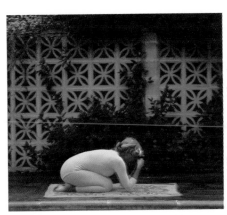

7 Returning to natural breathing for **7–9**, lower feet, knees and hips to ground. Sitting on heels, remain leaning forwards. Resting elbows in front of knees, place thumbs in eye sockets and relax to prevent dizziness.

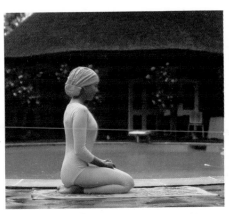

8 Slowly unfold to upright position with one hand resting in other, palms uppermost and tips of thumbs gently touching for few minutes.

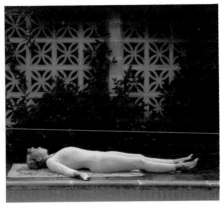

9 Relax into Resting Pose, lying on back with legs and arms comfortably arranged, eyes closed.

Yogatone continued

Breathing pattern Hold for Complete Breath at the end of every stage of the exercise.

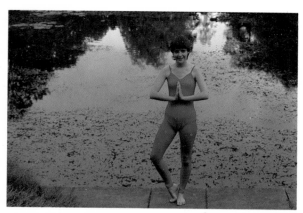

Tree Lotus: 1 Stand with legs together, arms at sides. Bring palms together at solar plexus. Raise right heel and press ball of foot against left heel. *Complete Breath*.

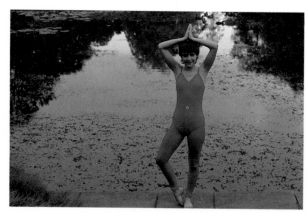

2 Arch right foot over onto toes, pushing heel forward and keeping supporting left leg straight. Raise hands to rest on crown of head, pressing elbows back. *Complete Breath*.

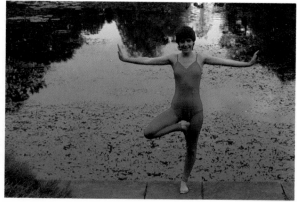

3 Draw right foot slowly up supporting leg until heel is tucked into groin in Tree Lotus position, lowering arms to shoulder level, palms pressing outwards. *Complete Breath*. Repeat, raising left leg.

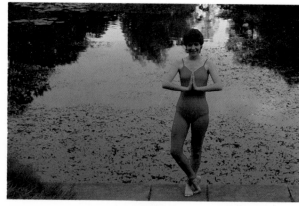

Half Stork Lotus: 1 Stand with legs together, arms at sides. Cross right foot over left, pressing down on ball of right foot, heel raised. Turn right knee outwards and bring palms together at solar plexus. *Complete Breath*.

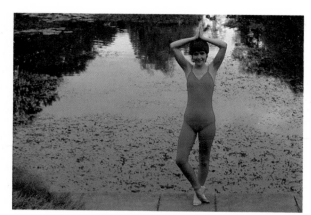

2 Arch right foot over onto toes, raising hands onto crown of head. Elbows should press back. *Complete Breath*. Lower arms to sides.

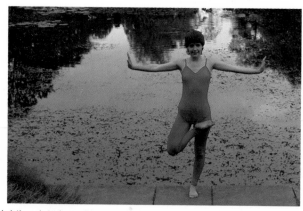

3 Holding right foot with both hands, thumbs to instep, lift up onto supporting left thigh, heel to groin, and balance with arms fully extended above head (palms together) or at shoulder level, palms pressed outwards. *Complete Breath*. Repeat, raising left leg.

Yogatone continued

Breathing pattern Normal (see page 17). No hold for Complete Breath.

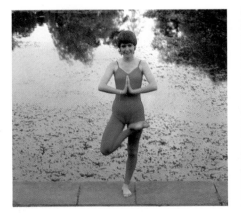

Complete Stork Lotus: 1 Continuing from Half Stork Lotus **3**, bring palms together at solar plexus and *inhale*.

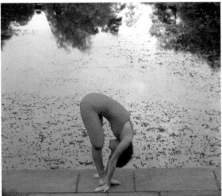

2 *Exhale*, folding head and torso forwards and down to place hands, palms downwards and fingers pointing backwards, on either side of supporting left leg.

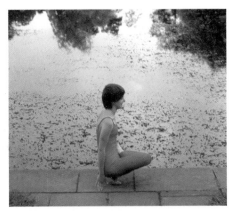

3 *Inhale*, squatting down to balance on supporting left heel, with right foot resting across left thigh and arms at sides, balancing on fingertips.

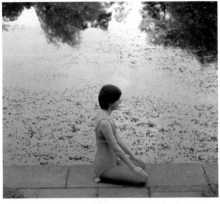

4 *Exhale*, sitting down on left foot, with right foot still resting across left thigh and hands resting on knees, palms downwards.

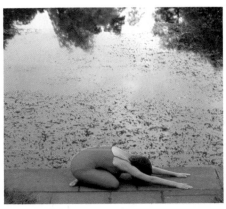

5 *Inhale*, sliding arms forward, chin towards ground. Hands should be in line with shoulders.

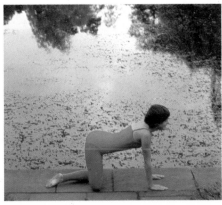

6 *Exhale*, raising hips until body rests on hands and knees at right angles to supporting limbs. Right foot now lies in front of left knee or on left thigh.

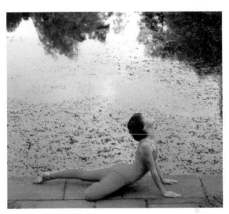

7 Still exhaling, lower body to ground, hips first. *Inhale*, arching head and torso back into Cobra (see page 42).

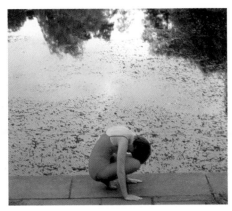

8 *Exhale*, pressing ball of left foot to ground and reversing hips up and back to squat shown in **3** by 'walking' hands backwards. Rest with forehead between knees and hands placed, palms downward, at sides.

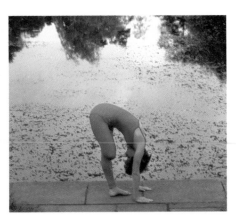

9 *Inhale*, tilting body forward and pushing hands down to straighten left leg and raise hips, unfolding to starting position. *Exhale*, lowering leg to ground. Repeat, raising left leg. Repeat whole sequence 1–10 times.

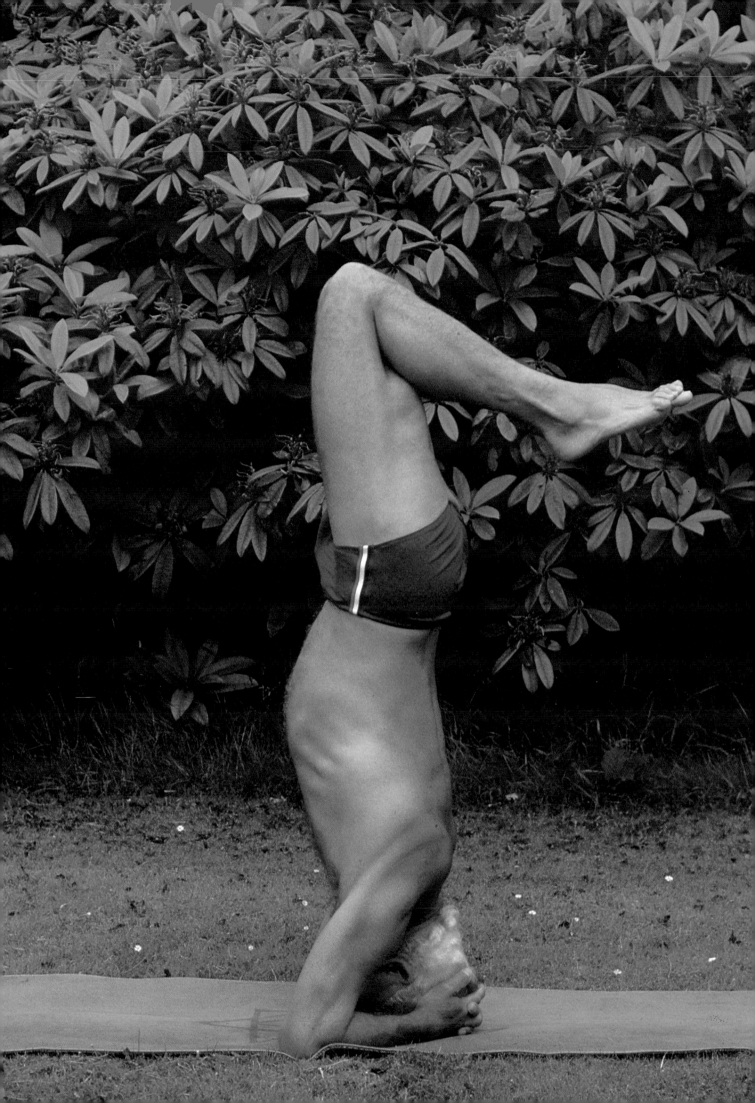

Getting Older
Ageing Limbs

With a history of minimal exercise behind you, you may well be feeling very nervous of beginning Yoga in your middle or later years. But, by using a wall for support and guidance, it is possible to regain the flexibility and confidence you enjoyed when younger.

Benefits You will increase the flexibility in your hips and waist with **1–3**, in your hips with **4–6**, and in your legs with **7–9**.

Breathing pattern Normal (see page 17).

Note At all stages remember to keep the whole of your back touching the wall. Try to make right angles with your torso or limbs as you perform the various bends and stretches. It is important to keep your weight evenly distributed between both feet throughout.

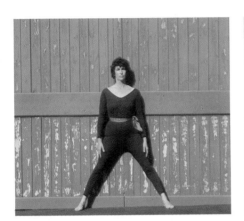

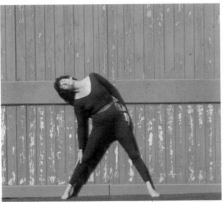

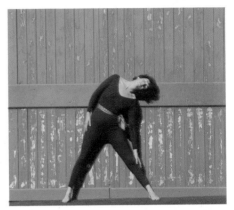

Triangle: 1 Stand against wall with legs 90–120cm (3–4ft) apart, toes in line with heels and arms at sides. *Inhale* 1–5, straightening spine up wall.

2 *Exhale* 1–5, relaxing to right side and sliding right hand down to calf. Body should remain flat against wall, feet unmoved, and chin off chest.

3 *Inhale* 1–5, straightening up. *Exhale* 1–5, relaxing to left side. Repeat 6 times on alternate sides.

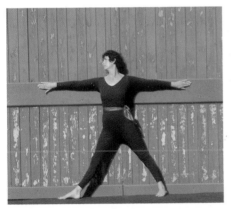

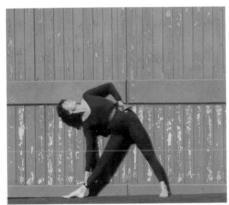

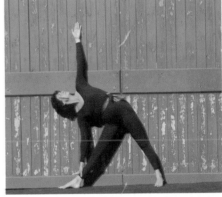

4 Stand as for **1**. *Inhale* 1–5, raising arms to shoulder level, palms facing backwards, and turning right foot to line up with centre of left foot, which is slightly inverted.

5 *Exhale* 1–5, stretching to right side and sliding right hand down leg, ideally to touch ground behind right foot. Left hand pulls left hip square to wall and head turns away from stretch, chin off chest.

6 *Inhale* 1–5, raising left arm over head so arms form vertical line. *Exhale* 1–5. *Complete Breath*, looking along raised arm. Straighten up, bringing left arm down to side. Repeat **4–6**, stretching to left.

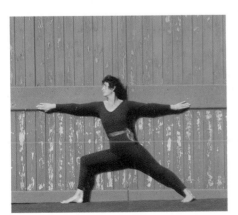

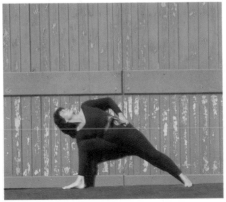

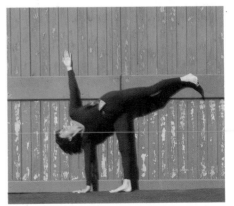

7 Return to position shown in **4**. Bend right knee to form right angle, thigh horizontal and knee above ankle. Open legs little wider if necessary.

8 *Exhale* 1–5, stretching down right thigh and slowly working right hand downwards from knee to ground behind foot as left hand pulls left hip square to wall and head turns away from stretch, chin off chest.

9 *Inhale* 1–5. *Exhale* 1–5, sliding right palm along ground in line with toes, straightening right leg, and raising left arm to form vertical line. *Complete Breath*. Bend right leg, returning to **4**. Repeat **7–9**, bending left leg.

Baldness

The Headstand is often called the 'King of all Yoga Exercises' and its benefits are, as one might expect, manifold. Initially, however, this position helps increase the blood supply to the head, and thereby to the scalp and hair and thus promotes hair growth through the pressure and release action of the exercise.

Other benefits The Headstand ensures health and vitality for the brain as well as the pituitary gland, relief from insomnia, tension, nervousness and anxiety, coughs, tonsilitis, bad breath, palpitations, constipation, asthma, bronchitis and poor circulation.

Note Many people imagine that the Headstand is well outside their capabilities. It's not nearly as difficult as it might appear to be and may be learned at any age. As always, the important thing is to go cautiously. Never push yourself further than feels comfortable.

Important See Health Precautions on page 12.

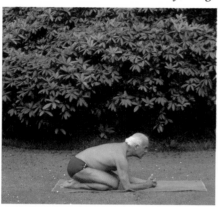

Triangle Headstand: 1 Sit on heels, toes together, knees apart, arms at sides. Bend head and torso forward to rest forearms on ground, elbows touching knees. *Inhale* 1–5.

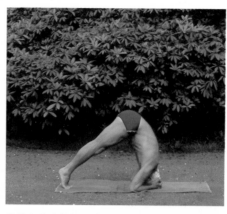

2 *Exhale* 1–5, lowering crown of head to ground, cupping head in hands, and raising hips, pushing up from knees and then balls of feet, weight balanced on hands, forearms and head.

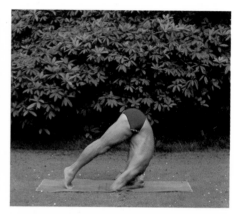

3 *Inhale* 1–5, drawing legs towards body, leaning weight over clasped hands, and keeping chin free from chest.

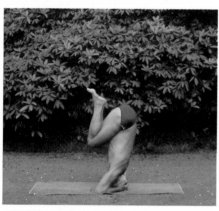

4 *Exhale* 1–5, contracting knees to body and heels to thighs, body now upright from head to hips, weight balanced on triangular base of arms and head.

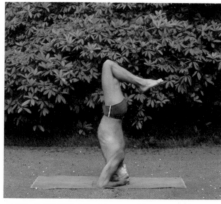

5 *Inhale* 1–5, arching back and raising knees with heels to contracted buttocks until directly above head. Open body by pushing elbows to ground from shoulders.

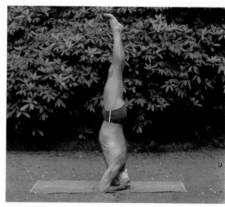

6 *Exhale* 1–5, unfolding legs until upright and slightly contracting hips and ribcage. *Complete Breaths*.

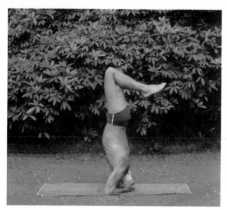

7 *Inhale* 1–5 and bend knees, heels moving towards buttocks as in **5**.

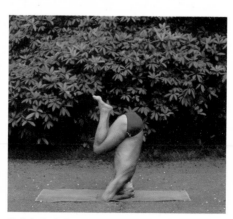

8 *Exhale* 1–5, contracting knees into chest and then gently lowering feet to ground.

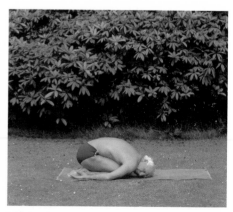

9 Returning to natural rhythm of breathing, lower knees to ground and hips to heels. Relax for a few minutes with one cheek to ground and arms at sides, palms uppermost. Repeat whole sequence 1–5 times.

Deafness

Everyone experiences some degree of deafness in a lifetime so it is comforting to know that there are exercises we can do to defer its advent. It also obviously makes sense to avoid constant loud noises, which will only wear out the ear drums.

Mantras These are sounds sometimes used to help people who find meditation difficult. Instead of practising inner visualization of objects (see page 87), they are encouraged to chant the chosen mantra out loud or internally, like humming a tune under your breath. The technique is also recognized to have physical benefits, and there are two special mantras designed to help the ears, eyes and throat. Sit in one of the Lotus positions (see page 37) or in a comfortable chair and chant either of the following sounds for 2–3 minutes each day: HAM or HRAH. *Inhale* deeply, and *exhale*, using your chosen mantra, feeling the vibration of the last sound.

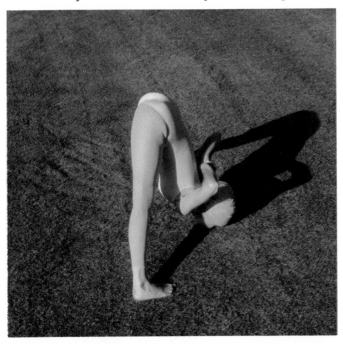

Pendulum: 1 Stand with legs 90–150cm (3–5ft) apart, heels slightly outwards and arms at sides. *Inhale* 1–5 and *exhale* 1–5, bending head and torso downwards and holding calves to pull ribs between straight legs, chin to ground. Press palms together or hold elbows behind back. *Complete Breath.*

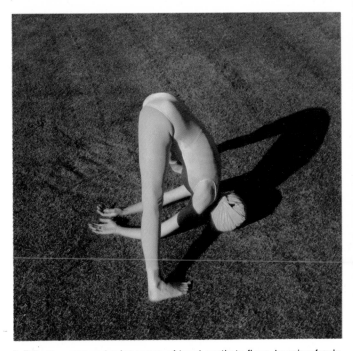

2 Release arms and relax crown of head gently to floor, hanging freely from hips between legs with arms really relaxed. *Complete Breaths.* Slowly unfold to upright position, arms at sides. Repeat **1–2** 6 times.

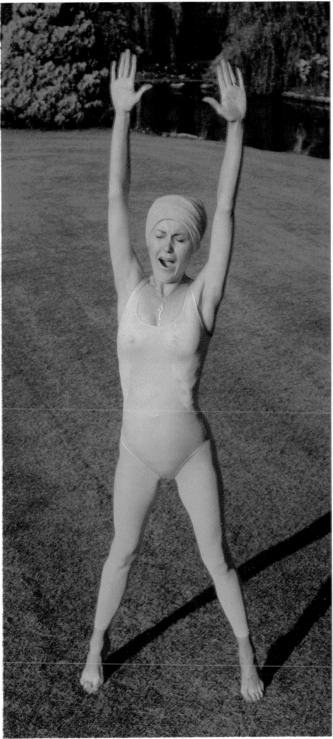

Yawning Stand with feet 60–90cm (2–3ft) apart, arms at sides. Stretch up onto toes, raising arms straight up over head and yawn several times. Relax, lowering arms to sides. Repeat 6 times.

Weak Eyesight

The muscles behind the eyes are known to deteriorate with advancing age, but with regular daily exercise good eyesight can be prolonged and weak eyes can be improved. These simple eye movements strengthen the eye muscles and improve your powers of concentration at the same time. It's never too young to begin them. The Cobra (page 42), the Bow (page 43), and all the balancing exercises are also excellent movements for strengthening the eye muscles.

Note Try to use your eyes as much as possible while doing other Yoga exercises, following the natural line of the body. It also helps strengthen your eye muscles to practise without glasses or lenses.

Distancing: 1 Sit on comfortable, straight-backed, armless chair either in one of Lotus positions (see page 37) or with feet evenly placed, flat on ground. Relax one hand on lap, other outstretched with forefinger upturned at eye level.

2 Look at nose, forefingertip, and then as far into distance as possible. Reverse order: distance, fingertip, nose. Close eyes and rest. Repeat 5 times.

3 Repeat 2 with the other forefinger extended at arm's length and eye level.

4 Repeat, closing one eye.

5 Repeat, closing other eye.

Verticals and Horizontals: 1 Sit as for Distancing, arms relaxed on lap.

2 Keeping head facing straight forward, look right, centre, left, centre. Repeat 5 times.

3 Again without moving head, look up, centre, down, centre. Repeat 5 times.

Diagonals: 1 Sit as for Distancing, arms relaxed in lap.

2 Move eyes to right upper corner and then diagonally down to left lower corner and back to right upper corner. Repeat 5 times.

3 Modify movement, looking from left upper corner diagonally down to right lower corner and back. Repeat 5 times.

Circles: 1 Sit as for Distancing, arms relaxed on lap.

2 Move eyes in clockwise direction, making complete circle. Repeat 5 times.

3 Reverse movement, making circle in anticlockwise direction. Repeat 5 times.

Expansion: 1 Sit as for Distancing, arms relaxed on lap.

2 Close eyes, screwing them up tightly and then opening them as wide as possible, looking to farthest point in distance. Repeat 10 times.

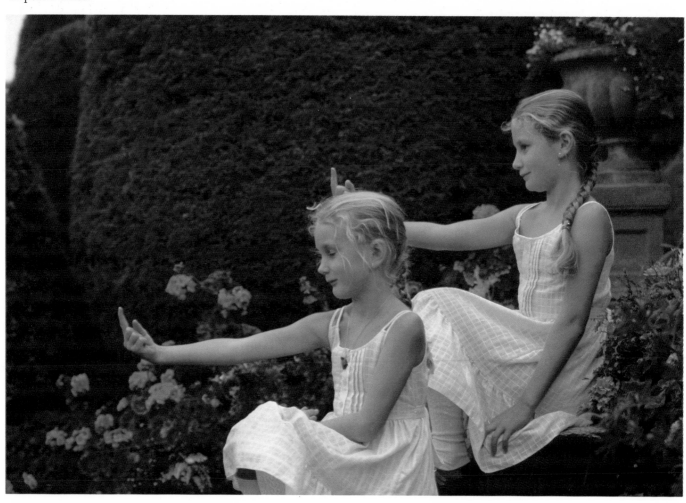

Keeping Warm

These movements can be done both in normal and cold conditions. Preparing the body for winter is as important as exercise once cold weather is upon us. If you can improve your circulation, you're helping to protect yourself against the problem of cold.

Note As with all the other sections of this book, the exercises should be accompanied by a properly balanced diet of fresh foods, including warming vegetable broths.

Warming Breath: 1 Sit comfortably, either in a chair, on a bed or on the floor, resting your hands on your lap, palms uppermost.

2 *Inhale* 1–3 through the nose. *Exhale* 1–3 through the mouth. Repeat in fairly quick succession 1–6 times.

3 Rest and return to your natural rhythm of breathing.

4 Perform 3 times daily: on rising, halfway through your day, and before retiring to bed.

Sun Breath: 1 Block left nostril with left thumb and *inhale* through right nostil for 5 counts.

2 Still blocking left nostril, clench left fingers into fist to close right nostril and hold breath for 5 counts.

3 Release left fingers and *exhale* for 5 counts through right nostril.

4 Repeat whole sequence 1–5 times.

Foot Warming Massages: Sit in comfortable chair and bend one knee, resting foot on opposite thigh. If this is difficult, sit on floor or in bed, bending foot towards you. Perform exercises 6 times on alternate feet.

Circles: Hold right foot with both hands and very slowly work thumbs in small circles over entire sole.

Vallies: 1 Draw thumb and forefinger of left hand down 'vallies' of right foot, i.e. forefinger down sole and thumb between tendons running from top of foot to toes.

2 End each stroke by gently pinching between toes.

Scissoring: 1 Holding right big toe with left hand and next toe with right hand, stretch one toe forwards, other backwards.

2 Reverse scissoring action 1–6 times.

3 Repeat, manipulating second and third toes in same way, and so on until all toes have been massaged.

Toe Circling: Hold each toe joint of right foot in turn with right thumb and forefinger and gently rotate with left forefinger and thumb in either direction.

Ankle Circling: Grasping right ankle between right thumb and fingers, apply circular press massage around ankle bones with thumb and fingertips.

Leg Warming: Foot crossovers: 1 Lie flat on back, arms raised to shoulder level, palm downwards, and place right heel between left big toe and second toe.

2 *Inhale* 1–3 and *exhale* 1–3, rocking over to left and lifting right hip off ground.

3 Repeat rocking to alternate sides 1–6 times. Relax.

4 Repeat sequence with left heel balanced on right foot.

Leg crossovers: 1 Lie on back, arms at shoulder level, palms downwards. *Inhale* 1–3, raising right leg.

2 *Exhale* 1–3, crossing right leg over left and lowering it towards floor on level with hips or shoulder.

4 *Inhale* 1–3, raising right leg.

5 *Exhale* 1–3, lowering right leg to starting position.

6 Repeat with left leg raised.

Knee Warming A: 1 Lying as for leg warming exercises, *inhale* 1–3, bending right knee. *Exhale* 1–3, crossing bent right leg over left leg, bending knee towards ground with foot resting on upper left thigh.

2 *Inhale* 1–3, raising knee and swivelling hip upright.

3 *Exhale* 1–3, opening bent right knee out to right side to touch ground, keeping foot free from left leg.

4 Repeat 1–6 times on alternate sides.

Knee Warming B: 1 Sit on ground or bed with legs forward and body supported by arms braced diagonally behind back.

2 *Inhale* 1–3, bending right knee.

3 *Exhale* 1–3, crossing bent knee over left leg to left side and simultaneously raising right hip.

4 *Inhale* 1–3, returning knee to upright position.

5 *Exhale* 1–3, lowering right knee to right side.

6 *Inhale* 1–3, raising right knee.

7 *Exhale* 1–3, lowering right leg to starting position.

8 Repeat on alternate sides 1–6 times.

Hip Warming: 1 Lying on right side, support head in right hand, elbow and upper arm to ground and left hand braced in front of solar plexus.

2 *Inhale* 1–3, raising left leg. *Exhale* 1–3, lowering leg to starting position. Repeat 1–6 times.

3 Reverting to natural breathing rhythm, raise left leg and move it backwards and forwards to touch ground behind and in front of body. Repeat 1–6 times.

4 Repeat on alternate sides 1–6 times.

Body Warming: Lie flat on back, arms resting on body or by sides, and wriggle body along ground in straight line by rolling hips from side to side. Repeat 6 times, travelling alternately forwards and backwards. Repeat movement in seated position, keeping legs straight and hands on thighs.

Arm and Finger Warming: Hold arms out in front at shoulder level, palms downwards. Stretch and contract fingers to form fists to maximum count.

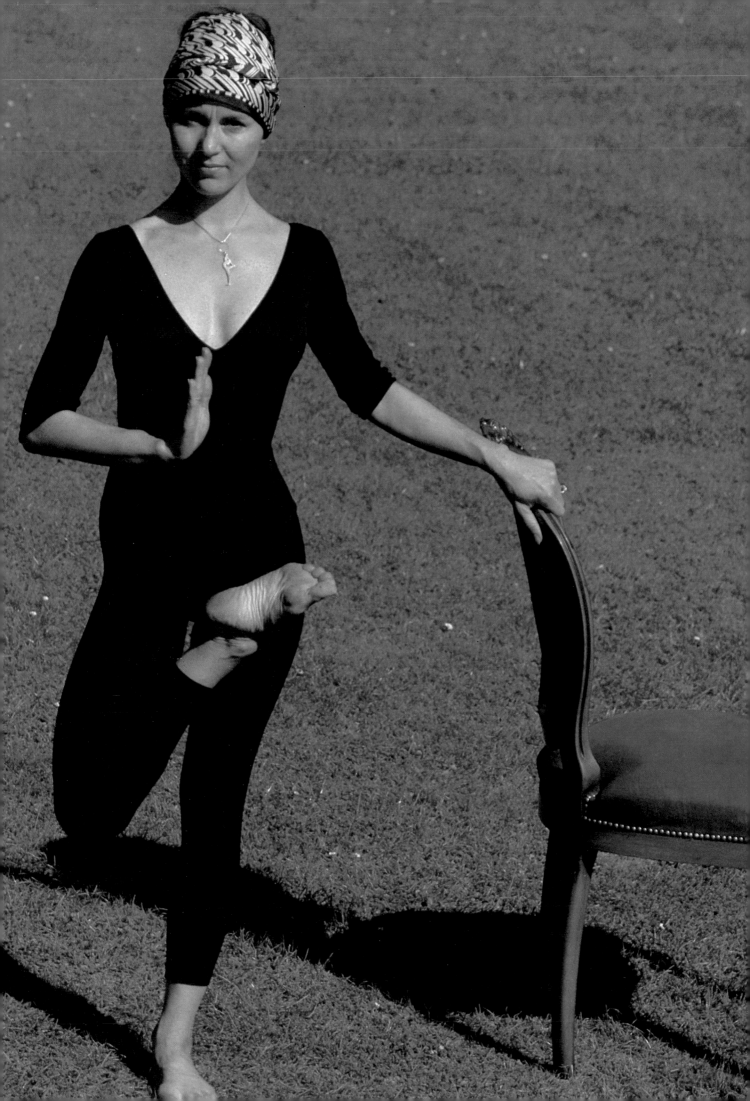

Disabled People

It has been my pleasure to teach and work with many disabled people. The experience has made me realize the potential of Yoga in this field.

The following exercises can be practised alone but, depending upon the severity of the handicap, some may need the help of a partner. Most can be practised standing, lying flat or seated on a chair. Choose whichever is most comfortable or appropriate.

Head: Beat head gently and rhythmically with tips of fingers for 2–3 minutes.

Scalp: 1 Press fingertips into scalp and inscribe small circles by pressing in a circular motion.

2 Massage whole scalp in same way.

Forehead: Stroke forehead with alternate palms, drawing right palm across from left to right and vice versa. Strokes should follow in fairly quick succession.

Face: 1 Starting on forehead, make small circular movements with fingertips to loosen the muscles.

2 Repeat until all face has been treated, apart from eyes.

Neck: 1 Place thumbs under chin and hands round neck, fingertips resting at base of skull. *Inhale* 1–5, lifting thumbs upwards to stretch tension out of neck. Hold 1–5.

2 *Exhale* 1–5, relaxing thumbs to return head to original position.

3 Repeat 1–5 times.

Shoulders A: 1 Interlace fingers, palms facing downwards. *Inhale* 1–5 and stretch arms forward and up over head, keeping fingers interlaced (and facing outwards) and contracting shoulders to ears.

2 *Exhale* 1–5, relaxing shoulders.

3 Repeat shoulder raising and lowering 1–5 times, inhaling as shoulders raised.

4 Release fingers and lower arms sideways to rest one palm on top of other, tips of thumbs touching.

5 Can also be performed with hands on lap, palms downwards.

Shoulders B: 1 Hold right elbow in left hand.

2 Forming fist with right hand, gently beat left shoulder 5–10 times.

3 Repeat with left fist to right shoulder. Keep the working wrist as relaxed as possible.

Chest A: 1 Place palms together at solar plexus. *Inhale* 1–5, turning hands to point fingers forwards (palms still pressing together), open arms and move them at shoulder level out to sides and round behind back (or chair if seated), trying to join hands. Hold 1–5.

2 *Exhale* 1–5, releasing hands and resting them on lap, one palm on top of other, tips of thumbs touching.

3 Repeat 1–5 times.

Chest B: Rub entire chest and ribcage with palms of hands in small up-and-down movements.

Breathing patterns I have indicated required breathing in certain exercises, based on principles described on page 17.

Waist: 1 *Inhale* 1–5, stretching right arm over head, palm facing front, fingers extended.

2 *Exhale* 1–5, sliding hand down back of neck.

3 *Inhale* 1–5, stretching spine upwards.

4 *Exhale* 1–5, side stretching (keeping raised arm in place) to left.

5 *Inhale* 1–5, returning to upright position.

6 Repeat sequence, stretching to right. Alternate side stretches 1–5 times.

Spine: 1 Sit on chair, hands resting on lap with left arm overhead. *Inhale* 1–5, stretching spine upwards.

2 *Exhale* 1–5 and twist to right, trying to grip chairback with one or both hands. Hold 1–5.

3 *Inhale* 1–5, returning to starting position.

4 *Exhale* 1–5, twisting to left.

5 Repeat on alternate sides 1–5 times.

Hips: Sit with hands resting on lap. Stretch arms over head, trying to grasp imaginary rope just out of reach with right, then left, hand. Breathe to natural rhythm.

Back: Lean forward and gently tap up and down back with under part of clenched fists, wrists relaxed.

Arms: 1 Clench right fist and gently tap up left inner arm from palm to armpit and down outside of arm from shoulder to back of hand.

2 Repeat 1–5 times on alternate arms.

Fingers and Toes: 1 Slide right fingers upwards between toes of left foot, pressing palm against sole.

2 Squeeze hand lightly. Hold 1–5 seconds.

3 Release and repeat on right foot with left hand.

Legs: 1 Forming hands into fists, gently tap down inside of legs to feet.

2 Continue movement up outside of legs to upper thighs.

3 Repeat sequence 1–5 times.

Butterfly Breath: 1 Start with arms relaxed by sides or on lap. *Inhale* 1–5, raising arms sideways up over head until backs of extended hands touch.

2 *Exhale* 1–10, slowly lowering arms to starting position.

3 Relax for few counts of natural rhythm of breath.

4 Repeat exercise 1–5 times.

Multiple Sclerosis

Many of the exercises on the previous page will ease and/or tone up your body and, since a lot of them can be performed standing, sitting or lying down, you can plan an exercise programme to suit your own needs.

In the early stages of this illness these chair exercises have proved to be most helpful to students I have taught. The chair has the obvious advantage of offering confidence and support. Look too at the simple body stretches described at the end of the Breathing and Relaxation section (page 17) and try the various massages described on pages 23 and 61.

Note Depression is quite naturally a frequent condition amongst sufferers, and all the breathing and meditation exercises mentioned elsewhere in this book will be of benefit.

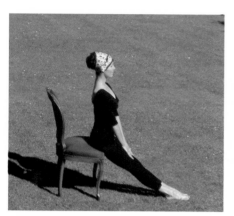

Jack Knife: 1 Sit on edge of chair, straight legs together and hands resting on thighs. *Inhale* 1–10.

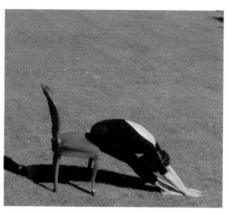

2 *Exhale* 1–10, sliding hands, head and torso down legs, keeping chin free from chest.

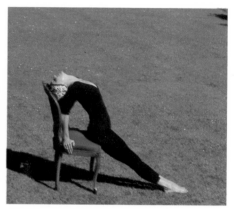

Cobra Repeat Jack Knife **1–2** but *inhale* 1–10 and unfold from hips to arch head backwards, bracing hands at sides of chair. *Exhale* to upright position. Repeat 5 times, raising hips so body forms diagonal line in final Cobra.

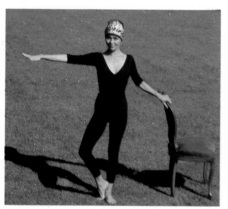

Half Stork Lotus: 1 Stand with legs together sideways to chair, holding chairback with left hand. Rest ball of right foot at right angles to left ankle, right arm, palm downwards, at shoulder level. Curl right toes to touch left heel.

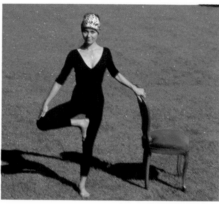

2 Slide right foot upwards to inside of left thigh by holding foot with right hand and then balancing with right hand on right knee. Hold position with right hand in Lotus position (see page 62) at solar plexus.

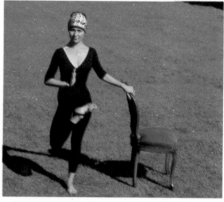

3 Cross right leg to rest, sole uppermost, at left groin, pushing right thigh outwards and hips forwards. Relax to Rag Doll position (see page 19), slowly unfolding, and repeat **1–3** on other side.

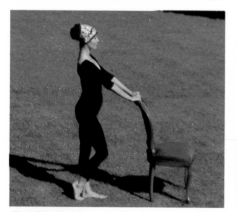

First Standing Pose: 1 Stand with legs together behind chair, holding onto its back. Bending right knee slightly, rest ball of right foot close behind left foot. *Inhale* 1–10.

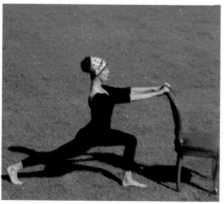

2 *Exhale* 1–10, lunging right leg backwards while trying to keep weight evenly distributed between both feet. Repeat **1–2** with left leg.

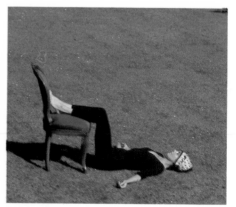

Resting Pose Lie on back with legs resting on chair seat, arms free from body and knees directly above hips. *Complete Breaths.*

Rheumatism and Arthritis

This series of hand exercises can be enjoyed by old and young alike. Extend your arms straight out in front of you so that your elbows and wrists are in line at shoulder level. The exercise for chilblains (on page 41) will also help those with rheumatism or arthritis in the feet.

For more comprehensive body stretching and strengthening techniques, turn back to the simple stretches described at the end of the Breathing and Relaxation section (see page 17). All of these are helpful and most are probably w range.

Note The last three movements are forms of m yourself or ask someone to help. In all massage natural oil, such as peach nut or apricot oil, for

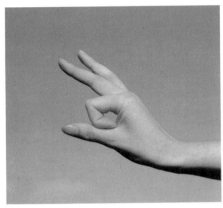

Curling Keeping free fingers fully extended, curl forefinger inwards, holding position with straight thumb. Repeat with each finger in turn. Repeat cycle 6 times with each hand.

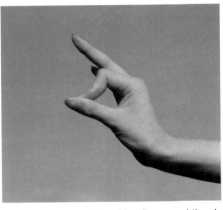

Contracting Press tips of forefinger and thumb together until first joint of forefinger bends inwards. Repeat, pressing each finger in turn onto thumb. Repeat cycle 6 times with each hand.

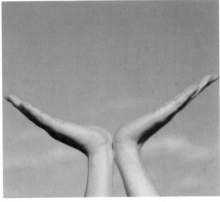

Fanning Press palms together at solar plexus. Slowly open fingertips and then palms outwards. Continue movement by pressing elbows together and opening wrists. Repeat 6 times.

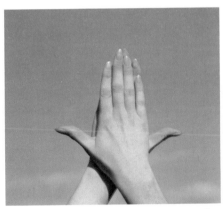

Fish Place one hand on top of other, palms downwards and fingers fully extended. Rotate thumbs in clockwise and then anticlockwise direction. Repeat 6 times.

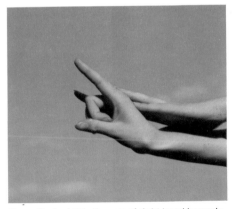

Deer Curl middle fingers of right hand inwards, holding position with thumb, while first and fourth fingers extend to form ears. Stroke deer's head with left hand. Repeat 6 times with each hand.

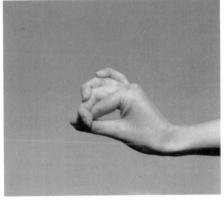

Peacock's Tail Press tips of right forefinger and thumb together. Using left hand to help, curl second finger over first joint of forefinger, third finger over second joint of second finger, and so on. Repeat 6 times with each hand.

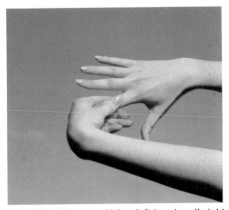

Stretching Massage Using left hand, pull right forefinger gently but firmly from base joint to fingertip, keeping other fingers fully extended. Repeat with each finger in turn. Repeat cycle 6 times with each hand.

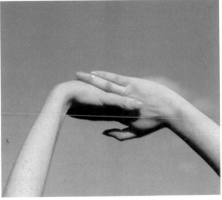

Valley Massage Fully extending fingers of right hand, draw thumb and forefinger of left hand firmly down 'valleys' between fingers, thumb pressing back of hand, forefinger pressing palm. Repeat cycle 6 times with each hand.

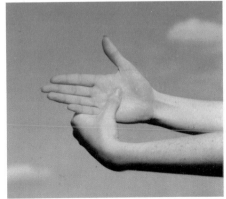

Rotating Massage Rotate tip of left thumb over entire surface of right palm, supporting hand with rest of fingers. Repeat massage on back of right hand. Repeat 6 times with each hand.

This simple mime was inspired by the lovely lotus lily which blossoms on a long green stem above the mountain waters of the Himalayas. It offers an imaginative and enjoyable way of exercising and strengthening your hands, wrists, and arms.

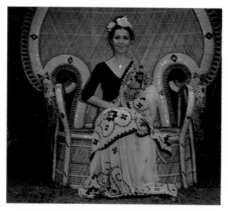 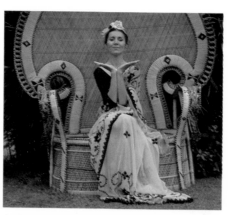 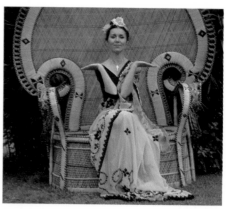

Lotus Hand Dance: 1 *The lotus starts its day in bud.* Sit on chair with legs together and palms together in First Lotus Hand Position at solar plexus.

2 *As the sun comes up so the petals open.* Move hands slowly upwards, bringing elbows together and opening palms outwards at shoulder level.

3 *By midday the lotus has opened its face completely to the sunshine.* Continue outward movement, opening wrists while keeping elbows together.

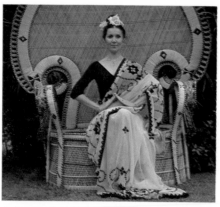 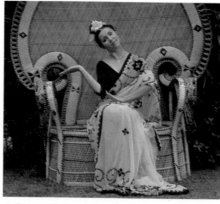 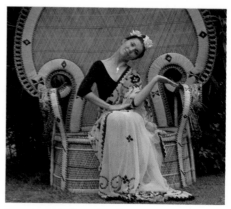

4 *It draws in light and strength through its petals to the stem and roots.* Draw both arms slowly downwards, bringing wrists and then fingertips together until heels of hands arch outwards, resting above thighs.

5 *The gentle breeze sways the plant, first to one side . . .* Gently slide right arm upwards and outwards, left hand sliding down right arm until fingertips touch right elbow, forming diagonal line from wrist to wrist.

6 *. . . then to the other.* Reverse movement to bring right hand back to left hand, straightening head (which mirrored hand movement), and then repeat sequence, sliding left arm upwards and outwards and inclining head to left.

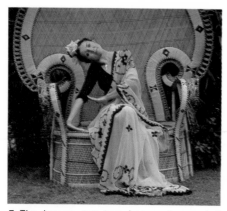 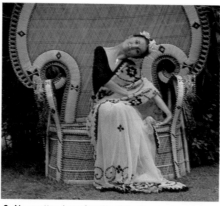 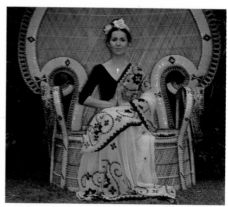

7 *The breeze can turn into a strong wind.* Reverse movement and repeat sequence to right, swaying farther still. Arching palm outwards, straighten right arm to touch seat with fingertips, pressing palm into inverted stretch.

8 *No matter how far the little flower bends . . .* Slide left hand down right arm to touch fingertips; inclining body to left, slide left arm upwards and outwards and straighten it to repeat inverted stretch as in **7**.

9 *. . . it always manages to keep control, returning to its original position.* Slide right hand down left arm until fingertips touch. Sway body back to centred, upright position, palms together at solar plexus.

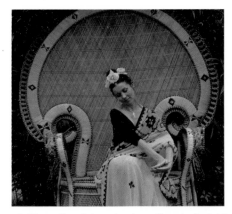

10 *Many tiny fish swim in a figure of eight around the roots.* Placing palm of straightened right arm on back of left hand, inscribe figure of 8 in air on left side of body at knee level.

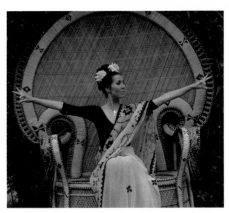

11 *All around there are tiny insects.* Curling both forefingers against thumbs, fully extend remaining fingers and raise straight arms on either side of body to shoulder level.

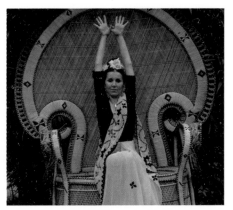

12 *They hover overhead.* Raise arms straight up over head, interlocking thumbs and waving other fingers backwards and forwards.

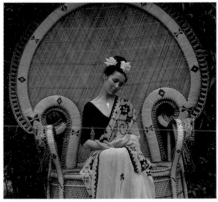

13 *The insects look down at the beautiful yellow flowers.* Lower arms sideways to rest one wrist upon another, palms uppermost, on thighs.

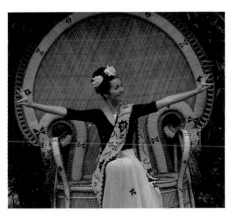

14 *All kinds of birds sing peacefully.* Raise straight arms on either side of body to shoulder level, with fully extended fingers splayed and thumbs touching extended forefingers.

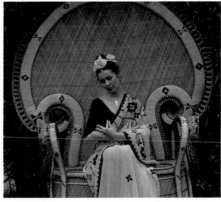

15 *Occasionally smaller birds land on the lotus lily to rest.* Lower both arms, curving them inwards and then round to rest splayed fingers inside curve of opposite elbow.

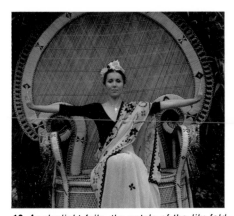

16 *As daylight fails, the petals of the lily fold upwards* . . . Straighten arms, raising them to shoulder level on either side of body and closing fingers and thumbs to press palms outwards.

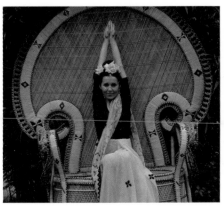

17 . . . *closing tightly to seal in the goodness of the day* . . . Continue upward movement of arms until they rest back to back above head.

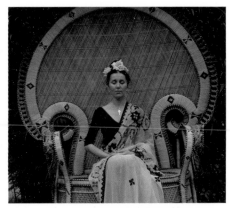

18 . . . *and resting peacefully until the dawn.* Slowly lower arms onto thighs, resting one hand in the other, palms uppermost, eyes peacefully closed.

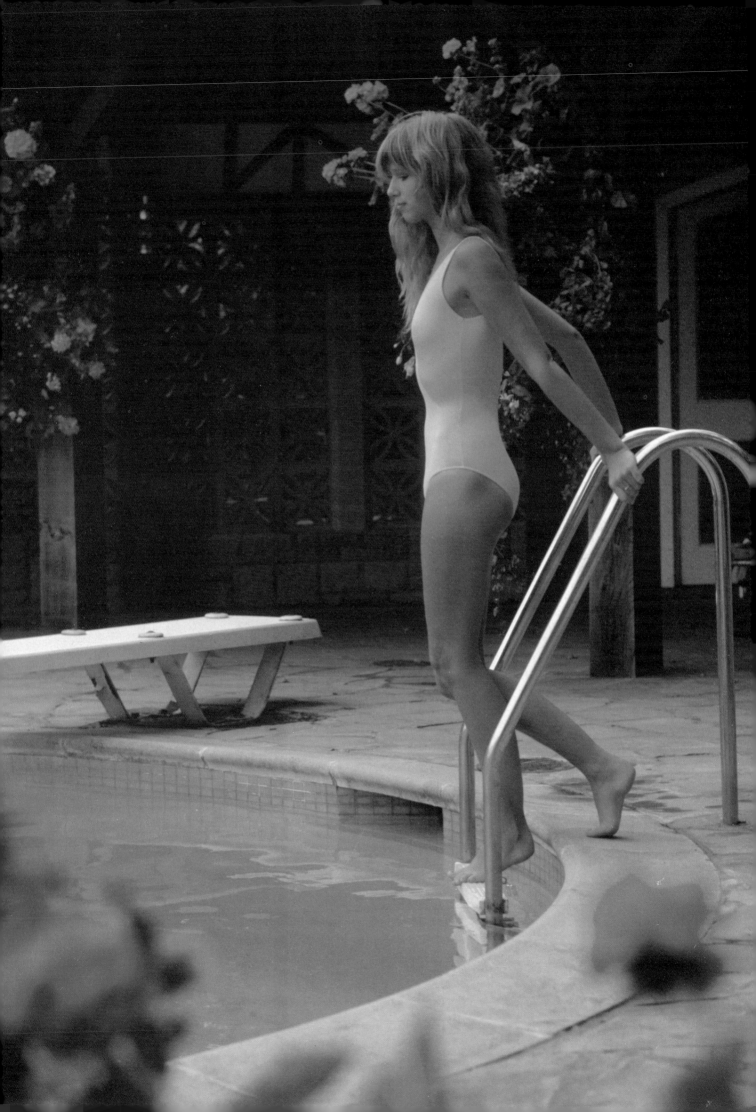

Yoga for Sport

It may seem curious to offer Yoga exercises for the sportsman or woman. We play games so aggressively – competing with ourselves, if not with others – and Yoga is essentially uncompetitive. In fact, however, Yoga's serene dynamics can offer very real benefits.

These exercises have been medically approved and are used to help prevent and even cure some of the ailments that beset people who play sport regularly. They are also an excellent way of stimulating your natural drive to improve your mental and physical powers.

Special benefits Turtle: stretches out tension in the spine and legs and strengthens body muscles. Cobra and Raven: strengthen arms and legs. Lunge: improves poise, balance and concentration.

Note for swimmers Before embarking on the Turtle, use the Plough (page 47) to stretch the back of your neck.

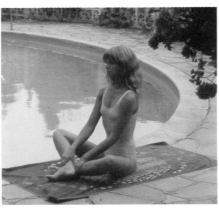

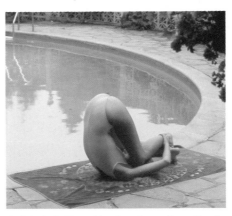

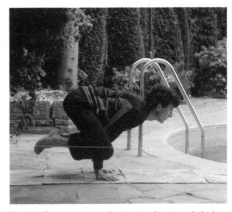

Swimmer: Turtle: 1 Sit with legs straight, feet together and arms at sides. Bending knees, cross ankles (right over left) and relax legs outwards, curling right foot round left with hands on ankles. *Inhale* 1–10.

2 *Exhale* 1–10, rocking legs forwards and backwards until right foot touches ground behind head, hands still clasping ankles.

3 *Inhale*, pushing away from ground with right foot. *Exhale* and, as spine touches ground, slide head between legs to lock feet round head. Release legs and rest on back with knees bent. Lower knees, sit up and repeat 1–10 times.

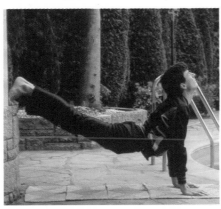

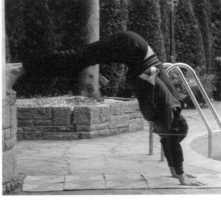

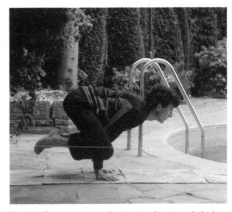

Boxer: Cobra: 1 Lie on stomach, arms at sides, legs straight and toes to wall. Place palms either side of head and 'walk' 60cm (2ft) up wall. *Inhale* 1–10 and fully extend arms under shoulders, arching head and torso backwards.

2 *Exhale* 1–10, pushing from shoulders to raise hips. Repeat, relaxing and raising hips 1–10 times (inhaling as relax, exhaling as stretch). Bend arms and walk down wall, lowering body to floor. Rest with head and arms to sides.

Raven Squat, arms between knees. *Inhale*, palms on ground. *Exhale*, tilting body forward to balance thighs against upper arms. Raise toes together and hold. Lower feet and rest, relaxed forward. Repeat 1–5 times.

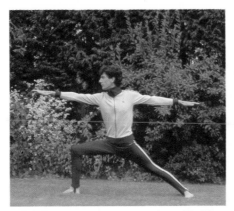

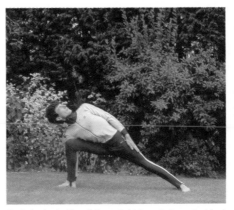

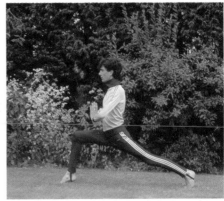

Fencer: Lunge: 1 Stand with legs 90–120cm (3–4ft) apart. Turn right heel to line up with left instep. Raise arms to shoulder level, turning head to right. *Inhale* 1–10, lunging to form right angle with right knee.

2 *Exhale* 1–10, sliding right hand down behind right leg to ground, bringing left arm down to side while keeping head up and looking along left shoulder. *Complete Breath*, weight evenly distributed.

3 *Inhale* 1–10, unfolding to **1**. *Exhale* 1–10, turning torso to right by pivoting on ball of left foot. Balance with palms together at solar plexus, raising and lowering right heel, body at constant height. Repeat, lunging with left leg.

Special benefits Squat Lotus: improves balance and poise, and strengthens legs and spine. Traction: reduces fat around waist, relieves fatigue, and strengthens ankle, knee and hip joints. Pigeon: develops poise, grace and balance, strengthens leg and arm muscles, and gives vertebral joints greater flexibility.

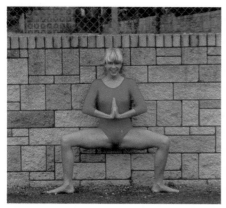

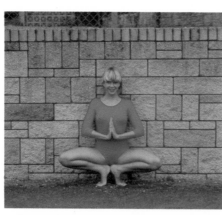

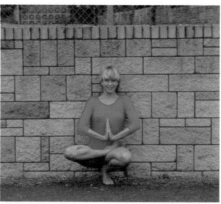

Horserider: Squat Lotus: 1 Stand against wall, legs 60–90cm (2–3ft) apart, arms at sides. Turn feet to side and *inhale* 1–10. *Exhale* 1–10, bending knees, palms together at solar plexus. *Inhale* 1–10, straightening up. Repeat 5 times.

2 Bring heels together. *Inhale* 1–10. *Exhale* 1–10, bending knees as for **1**, pressing outwards and resting on balls of feet. Repeat 5 times.

3 Raise right foot, sole upwards, onto left thigh, thumbs to instep. *Complete Breath*, palms together at solar plexus. Lower foot and rest, sitting on heels, hands on lap, palms uppermost, thumbs touching. Repeat, raising left leg.

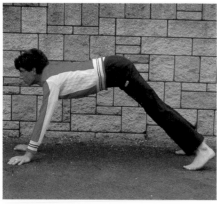

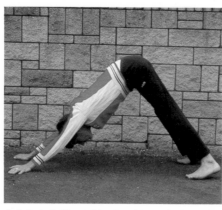

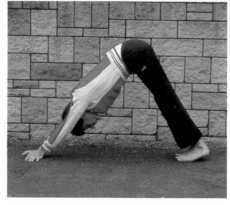

Golfer or Footballer: Traction: 1 Stand with feet 60–90cm (2–3ft) apart, arms at sides. Relax head and torso forward from hips. Rising on toes, 'walk' hands forward to rest just in front of shoulders. *Inhale* 1–10, chin away from chest.

2 *Exhale* 1–10, pushing head towards feet, with chin to ground and arms fully extended, working from shoulders. Legs should be straight, heels towards ground. Raise head and relax forward. Repeat **1–2** 5 times.

3 Repeat **1–2** with palms turned outwards, wrists touching and feet together. Kneel down and relax forwards with forehead to ground, arms at sides, palms downwards.

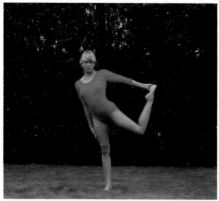

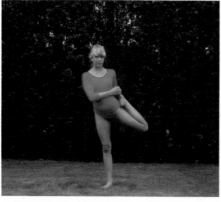

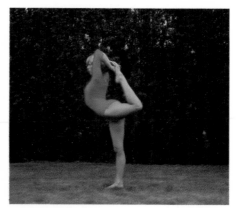

Gymnast: Lord of the Dance: 1 Stand with legs together, arms at sides. Bend left leg backwards and clasp toes in left hand. *Inhale* 1–10, stretching leg and arm sideways away from body to bring foot to shoulder level.

2 *Exhale* 1–10, pulling left toes into left side at waist or shoulder, holding foot with both hands.

3 Hold left big toe with right hand and *inhale* as raise right arm over head, arching head and torso backwards while left arm bends back under right arm to grasp foot. *Exhale*. Relax and repeat with right leg. Repeat **1–3**, kneeling.

Special benefits Hamstring: stretches and tones muscles, relieving stiffness in legs and hips, and making hips and spine more elastic; it also corrects weak wrists. Bridge: tones stomach and thigh muscles and makes spine more flexible. Bow: improves concentration and strengthens shoulders, arms and wrists.

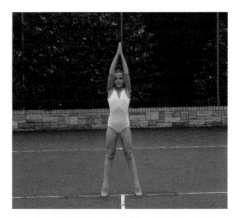

Tennis or Squash: Hamstring Stretch: 1 Stand with feet 60–90cm (2–3ft) apart. Bring palms together at solar plexus. *Inhale* 1–10, rising on-to balls of feet, palms over head. *Exhale* 1–10 and relax, arms to sides. Repeat 1–5 times.

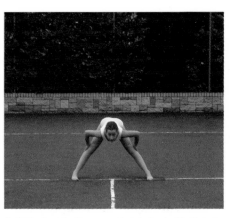

2 With feet farther apart, *inhale* 1–10. *Exhale* 1–10, relaxing head and torso downwards, hands behind knees. Turn heels outwards and stretch down, pulling ribs between legs, looking forward. Unfold upright. Repeat 1–5 times.

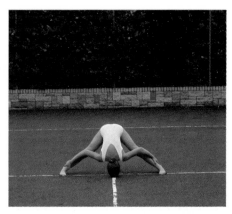

3 Widening space between feet again, slide hands farther down legs and repeat **2**, continuing downward stretch, bringing chin then crown of head to ground. *Complete Breath*. Unfold to upright position. Repeat 1–5 times.

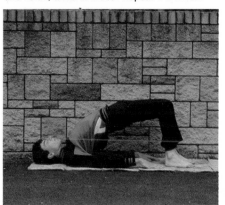

Sailor: Bridge: 1 Lie on back, legs together and arms at sides. Bend knees until raised above ankles. *Inhale* 1–10, raising hips, keeping knees and ankles together. *Exhale* 1–10, lowering hips to ground. Repeat 1–5 times.

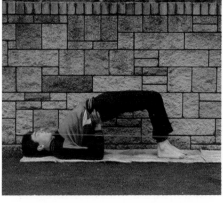

2 *Inhale* 1–10, raising hips. *Exhale* 1–10, placing hands under small of back, fingers outwards. *Complete Breath*. Relax on back, knees bent. Repeat 1–5 times. Relax, lying flat, and draw knees up to chest to rock from side to side.

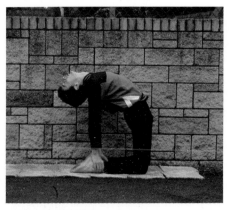

Camel Sit on heels, arms at sides. *Inhale* 1–10, raising hips. *Exhale* 1–10, arching head and and body back until hands clasp ankles or push into small of back. *Complete Breath*. Relax body and head forward. Repeat 1–5 times.

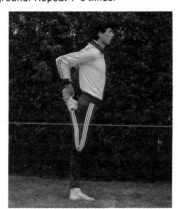

Archer: Bow: 1 Stand with feet together and arms at sides. Bend right foot up to buttocks and interlace fingers below toes, thumbs to instep. *Inhale* and *exhale*, pulling foot into small of back.

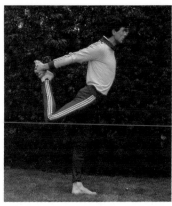

2 Move thumbs from instep, still grasping feet below toes. *Inhale* 1–10, pushing foot away from body, with shoulders contracted back and chest expanded. *Exhale* 1–10 and hold position for *Complete Breath*.

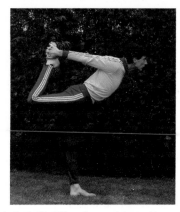

3 *Inhale* 1–10, tilting forward from hips while body still fully arched and arms extended. *Exhale* 1–10, returning to upright position. Repeat, raising left foot.

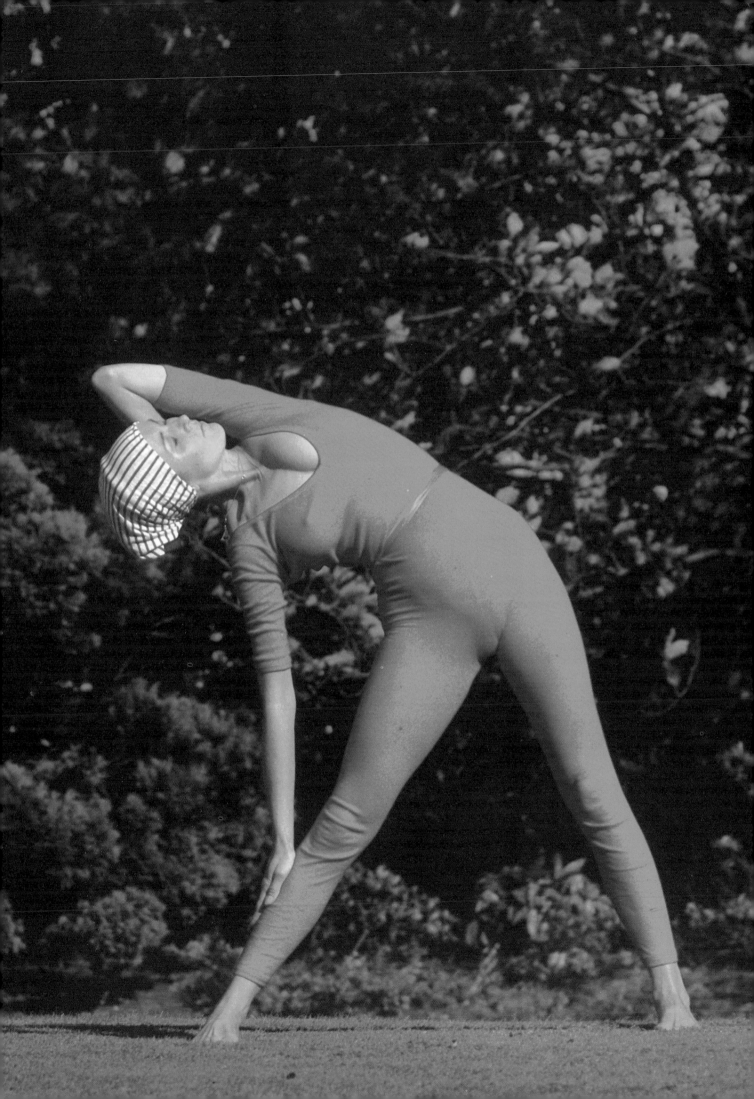

Planning Exercise Sequences
Yogarhythm

You may well have decided to use this book initially because it offered a solution to a health problem. As you become familiar with the basic concepts of Yoga and your problems begin to yield to a general sense of well-being, you'll probably feel the desire to create a broader, less specialized exercise schedule.

My Yogarhythm Series offer an interesting and modern approach. Each sequence has been choreographed to link classical Yoga movements together into a flowing rhythmical exercise programme. Many students who are perhaps not so agile or lack natural rhythm find it helpful to practise to a musical accompaniment. This example can be performed to 'Windmills of Your Mind'. See page 73 for more exercise sequences.

Note The series can be practised either alone or with a group of people forming a circle. In group work, join hands with your immediate neighbours for **6, 22,** and **32–33**.

Breathing pattern Normal (see page 17).

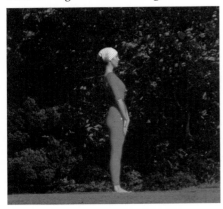

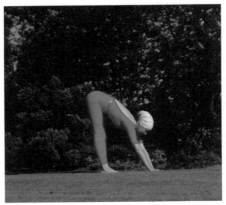

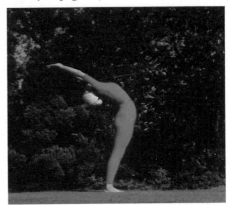

1 Stand with legs together and palms resting on thighs. *Inhale* 1–3.

2 *Exhale* 1–3, sliding palms down legs and along ground away from feet, keeping legs as straight as possible and chin away from chest.

3 *Inhale* 1–3, stretching upwards and arching backwards, while swinging arms slowly and simultaneously up, back and round to sides.

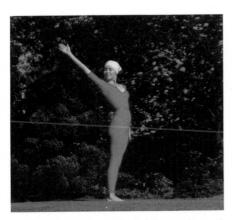

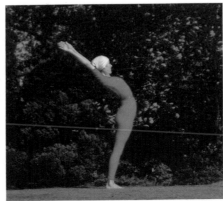

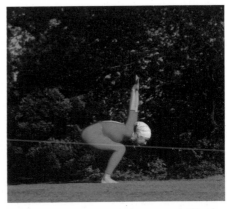

4 *Exhale* 1–3, 'windmilling' right arm forward, up, back and round to side, head following swinging hand throughout. Repeat with left arm.

5 *Inhale* 1–3, windmilling both arms forward, up and round to sides, head facing forward and body arching with movement.

6 *Exhale* 1–3, interlocking thumbs behind back, and bend knees at right angles to ground, pressing torso down onto thighs and raising joined hands straight up over shoulders.

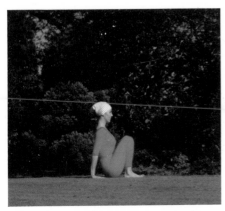

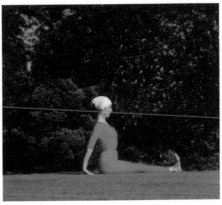

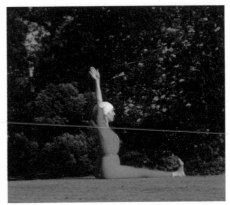

7 *Inhale* 1–3, lowering hands to ground, palms downwards behind and facing body, and then hips, keeping knees raised and together.

8 *Exhale* 1–3, sliding legs forward, keeping body erect and moving arms to either side of body, fingertips touching ground.

9 Facing front throughout, *inhale* 1–3, raising straight right arm sideways above head, and *exhale* 1–3, lowering arm down to ground, palm facing outwards. Repeat with left arm. *Inhale* 1–3 with arms at sides.

Yogarhythm continued

Breathing pattern Normal (see page 17).
Note Head should turn upwards under raised arm during stretches throughout remainder of sequence.

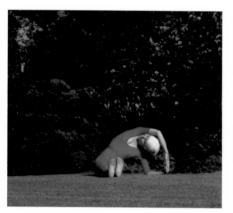

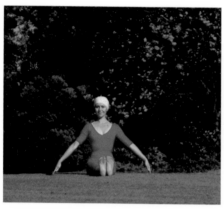

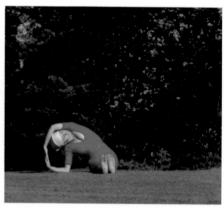

10 *Exhale* 1–3, stretching head, torso and hips to left side and resting left forearm on ground with palm turned at right angles to it, as right arm (palm uppermost) arcs over head and down to rest, palm to palm, on left side.

11 *Inhale* 1–3, recovering to upright seated position, straight arms extended on either side, palms inwards and fingertips touching ground.

12 *Exhale* 1–3, repeating sideways stretch shown in **10** to right, with left arm over head.

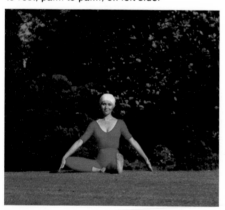

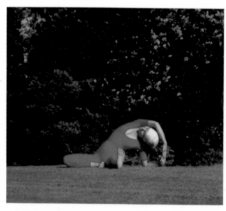

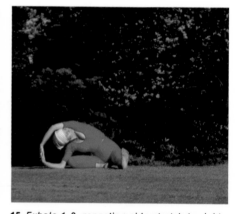

13 *Inhale* 1–3, recovering to upright seated position, arms extended at sides. *Exhale* 1–3, sliding both hands (left on right, palms downwards) down right leg, and *inhale*, drawing foot up to inner left thigh. Extend arms at sides.

14 *Exhale* 1–3, repeating side stretch to left, with right arm over head. *Inhale* 1–3, recovering to upright seated position, arms extended at sides.

15 *Exhale* 1–3, repeating side stretch to right, with left arm over head. *Inhale* 1–3, recovering to upright seated position, arms extended at sides.

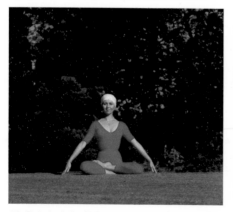

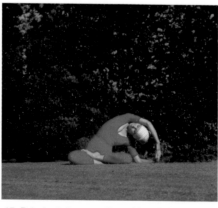

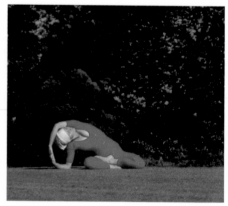

16 *Exhale* 1–3, sliding both hands down left leg, right hand on top of left, and draw extended left foot into one of Lotus positions (see page 37). *Inhale* 1–3, extending arms at sides.

17 *Exhale* 1–3, repeating side stretch to left. *Inhale* 1–3, recovering to upright seated position, arms extended at sides.

18 *Exhale* 1–3, repeating side stretch to right and folding left knee onto right knee once side stretch is achieved.

Yogarhythm continued

Breathing pattern Normal (see page 17).

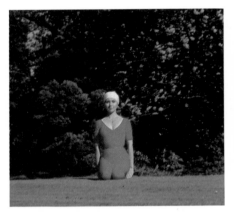

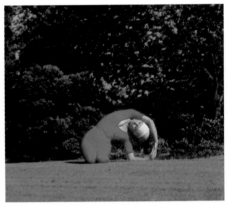

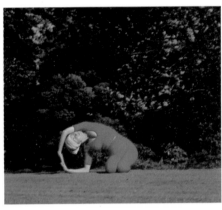

19 *Inhale* 1–3, swivelling onto knees and sitting back on heels. Extend arms at sides.

20 *Exhale* 1–3, repeating side stretch to left. *Inhale* 1–3, recovering to upright position, sitting on heels and arms extended either side.

21 *Exhale* 1–3, repeating side stretch to right. *Inhale* 1–3, recovering to upright position, arms extended at sides.

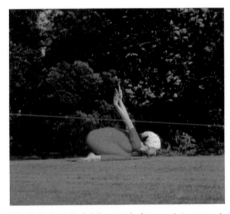

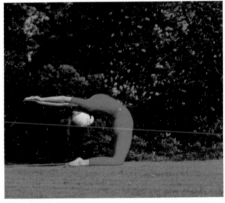

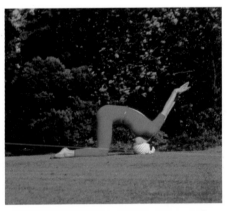

22 *Exhale* 1–3, folding body forward, torso onto knees, and raising straight arms up behind back as chin touches ground.

23 *Inhale* 1–3, raising hips and torso into kneeling position and swinging arms forwards, up and back to arch body with arms' natural swing.

24 *Exhale* 1–3, stretching head and torso forward, pushing over onto crown of head, and swinging arms down, round and behind back to interlock thumbs.

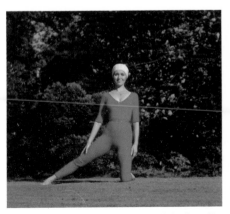

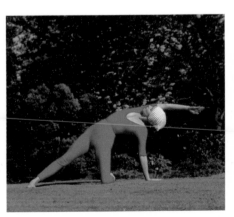

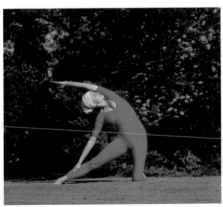

25 *Inhale* 1–3, unfolding to upright kneeling position, arms at sides. Extend right leg to side, turning toes to front in line with left knee.

26 *Exhale* 1–3, repeating side stretch to left, left palm flat on ground and right arm fully extended over head horizontal with ground. Keep body square to front. *Inhale* 1–3, recovering to upright position, arms at sides.

27 *Exhale* 1–3, stretching to right, sliding right palm down right leg, and extending left arm over head. Recover to upright position, knees together. Repeat **25–27**, extending left leg to side.

Yogarhythm continued

Breathing pattern Normal (see page 17).

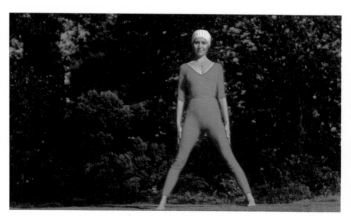

28 *Inhale* 1–3, rising to feet and moving left leg to side to stand with feet 60–120cm (2–4ft) apart, toes facing front.

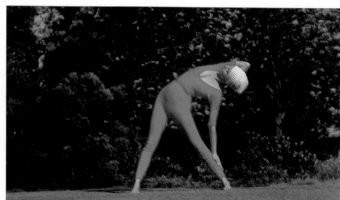

29 *Exhale* 1–3, stretching to left side, sliding left palm down left leg, and raising right arm over head before folding it down spine. *Inhale* 1–3, recovering to upright position, arms at sides.

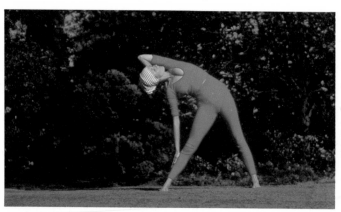

30 *Exhale* 1–3, repeating stretch to right side with left arm folded down spine. *Inhale* 1–3, recovering to upright position, bringing legs together and arms to sides.

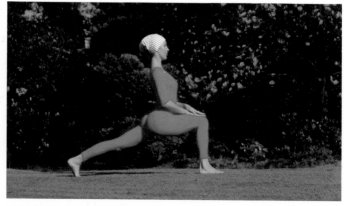

31 *Exhale* 1–3, sliding left leg backwards on ball of foot and bending right knee to form right angle. Rest palms on right knee, left on right. *Inhale* 1–3, windmilling arms forward, up, back and down to sides.

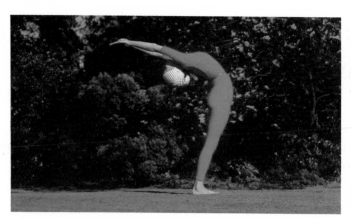

32 *Exhale* 1–3, drawing left leg forwards to rest beside straightened right leg. *Inhale* 1–3, arching head and torso backwards, windmilling arms with interlocked thumbs forward, up and back.

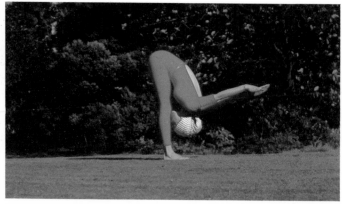

33 *Exhale* 1–3, bending head and torso forward and downward to touch legs, arms swinging down and up behind back, thumbs interlocking. *Inhale* 1–3, relaxing arms, hands beside feet. *Exhale* 1–3, slowly unfolding upright, hands on thighs.

Once you can perform this series confidently and without prompting, you'll begin to realize that Yogarhythm is a meditation in movement. And by practising daily a series of classical Yoga exercises you will soon be inspired to compile your own rhythmic sequences.

The following combinations of exercises are offered only as a basis for personal experiment. Exercises can be added or taken away according to your particular needs or inclination.

Combinations of exercises can also be performed in series.

You do not have to link your series to a musical background but it can give a new dimension to your practice. Each movement and/or breath can be linked to a musical tempo if you choose.

All these exercises should be performed on alternate sides. Breathe to your own natural rhythm, to the counts given in the various sections of the book, or to a musical tempo.

Standing

1. First Standing Pose
   page 44
1. Shoulder Stretch
   page 21

2. Tree Lotus
   page 50
2. Standing Twist
   page 20

3. Half Stork Lotus
   page 50
3. Rag Doll
   page 19

Balancing

1. Standing Bow
   page 67
1. Triangle Headstand
   page 54

2. Raven
   page 65
2. Bridge
   page 67

3. Headstand
   page 49
3. Pose of Tranquillity
   page 27

Head to Toe Stretch

1. Eye Circles
   page 56
4. Arm Circles
   page 69 **(1–5)**

2. Head Roll
   page 21
5. Triangle
   page 53

3. Shoulder Roll
   page 21
6. Pendulum
   page 55

Kneeling

1. Cat
   page 44

2. Camel
   page 67

3. Neck and Shoulder Stretch
   pages 21–22

Seated

1. Seated Squat
   page 30

2. Preparation for Lotus
   page 37

3. Full Lotus
   page 37

Side Stretch

1. Hip Warming
   page 57

2. Seated Side Stretch
   page 70 **(10–12)**

3. Rotation Squat
   page 30

Lying on Stomach

1. Cobra
   page 42

2. Locust
   page 44

3. Bow
   page 43

Lying on Back

1. Knee to Ear Pose
   page 26

2. Turtle
   page 65

3. Hug
   page 44

Lying on Shoulders

1. Bridge
   page 67

2. Plough
   page 47

3. Shoulder Stand
   page 48

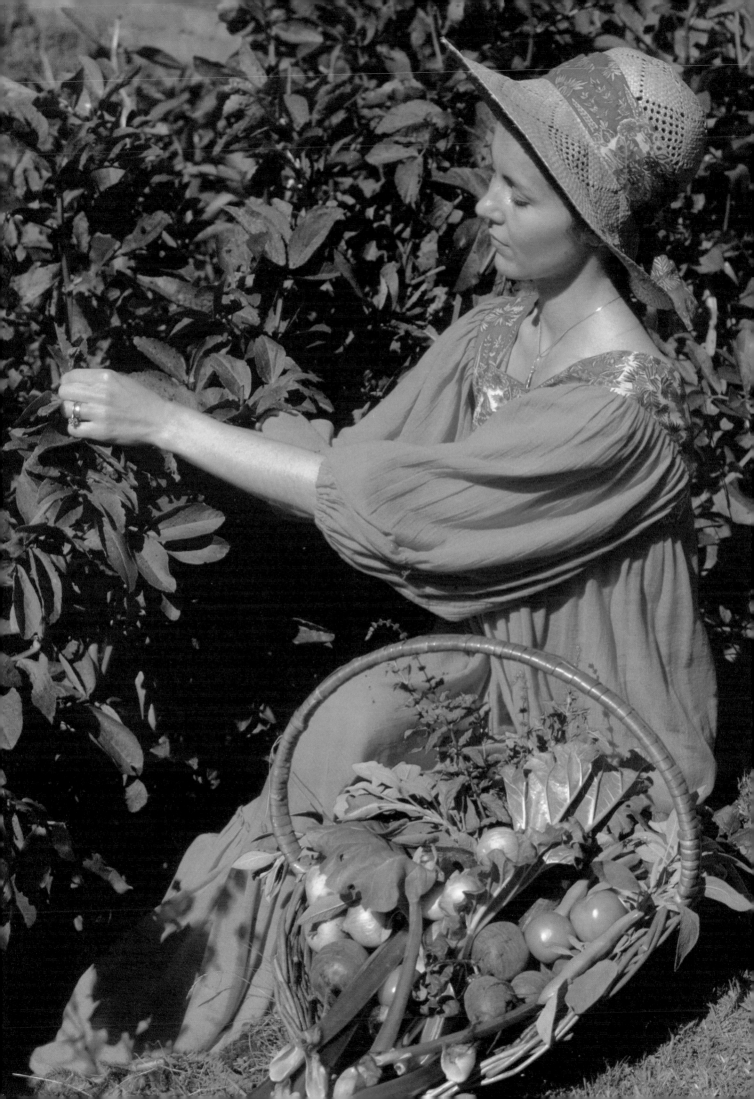

Eating for Health

The key to a lifetime's sensible eating is to choose the foods which suit *your* body's needs. The first step is to understand basic food values and learn what constitutes a balanced meal. The second is to consider your own lifestyle, your temperament, your finances. Obviously what suits Jane, a 16-year-old competitive swimmer, isn't going to be right for Sam, who's nearly 60 and does a desk job.

Basic food values

Dieticians, doctors and scientists tell us that our food must contain certain health-giving constituents if our bodies are to function properly. Any good book on nutrition will explain in detail what the body's requirements are. Establishing and maintaining a balanced diet means making sure that your eating habits provide you daily with all the required nutrients. But as a simple guide to the basics of good eating, you'll be doing fine if you make sure that every meal contains at least one example from each of the groups of health-giving constituents listed below.

Protein is essential for growth and the repair of body tissue. It is as important to the elderly as to the young child. Protein is the big hunger satisfier.

Found in dairy products, soya beans, root vegetables, nuts, pulses, wholegrain cereals, wholemeal flour and bread, meat, fish and poultry.

Vitamins help to build and mend body tissues. The principle vitamins are as follows:

Vitamin A for fighting disease	Found in dairy products (eggs, milk, butter and cheese), vegetable margarine, leafy and green vegetables, carrots, watercress, celery, endives, tomatoes, prunes, dried apricots and figs, oranges, meat, especially liver and lamb.
Vitamin B for healthy muscular and nervous systems/ utilization of carbohydrates	Found in wholemeal bread and flour, brazilnuts, peanuts, lentils, leafy and green vegetables, soya beans, yeast, dairy products, liver, yogurt, oatmeal.
Vitamin C for vitality/building and mending body tissues	Found in citrus fruits, other fresh fruit (especially blackcurrants), tomatoes, potato jackets, spinach, leafy and green vegetables, watercress, peppers, cauliflower.
Vitamin D for healthy teeth and bones	Found in eggs, vegetable margarine, butter.

Carbohydrates provide heat and energy for physical and mental exertion by supplying immediate calories. They also help the process of assimilation and digestion. These are the starchy, sugary foods. If you're over-indulgent here, you'll have weight problems. The other danger is in eating over-refined carbohydrate products, such as white bread, white sugar, sweets, cakes, ice cream, drinks and so on. In their natural forms wheat and sugar are perfectly balanced foods. It is in the making of white flour or sugar that most of the vitamins and minerals are removed, sometimes (ironically) to be placed by 'added vitamins'. Go for wholemeal bread (which uses the whole grain – the germ, the starch and the bran) and for honey or the more natural dark brown sugar. The best carbohydrates are as follows.

Found in root vegetables, fruits (both dried and fresh), wholemeal flour and bread, wholegrain cereals, honey and dark brown sugar.

Fats feed the nervous system as well as generally lubricating our skin and building a protective layer against cold weather. As with all the essential constituents of a balanced diet, we should be sensible about how much of them we eat. Lavish amounts of any food, however good, will cause an imbalance which prevents the correct functioning of the body, and fats are no exception. The debate about the wisdom of eating animal fats and their possible connection with heart disease still continues. I list below the most natural fats. All but milk are vegetable based. Low-fat milks are now commonly available if required.

Found in vegetable oils and margarine, milk, nuts, avocados.

Minerals perform a variety of vital tasks, many of them in conjunction with vitamins.

Calcium for strong teeth and bones/healthy blood	Found in milk, cheese, eggs, almonds, brazilnuts, green and leafy vegetables, wholemeal bread and flour, potatoes, soya flour, oatmeal, dried apricots, citrus fruits, celery, parsley, figs, rhubarb, blackberries.
Phosphorus also for sound bones and teeth/healthy blood	Found in almonds and other nuts, cereals, grapes, citrus fruits, blackberries, cranberries, cucumbers, wholemeal bread and flour, wheat germ, soya beans, tomatoes, watermelons.
Iron for vitality/healthy blood	Found in eggs, cheese, pulses, soya, lentils, wholemeal flour and bread, wheatgerm, oatmeal, yeast, black treacle, plain chocolate, nuts, dried fruits, tomatoes, bananas, green and leafy vegetables, dried beans and peas.

Copper for absorption of iron	Found in fresh and dried fruit, green and leafy vegetables.
Iodine for healthy thyroid gland	Found in fish, green and leafy vegetables, carrots, cucumbers, prunes, tomatoes, radishes, pineapples.
Potassium for muscle building/healthy liver	Found in nuts, fruit, green and leafy vegetables.
Sodium for digestion/elimination of carbon dioxide	Found in wholemeal bread and flour, celery, bananas, green and leafy vegetables, beetroot, rye bread.
Chlorine for cleansing/expelling waste matter/purifying blood	Found in fruits, vegetables.
Sulphur purifies blood/aids healthy digestion/prevents toxic build-up	Found in fruits, vegetables.

All these lists may appear rather overwhelming at first but remember: most foods contain more than one form of nutrient. If you make sure you plan your eating around lots of *fresh* fruit and vegetables, high-protein foods (like cheese, eggs, meat in small quantities, nuts and milk), with small amounts of carbohydrates and fats, you'll be having a sensible, well-balanced diet.

It is not essential, as many people think, to turn vegetarian and eliminate all animal products from the diet to be really healthy. For many people vegetarianism may not suit either their lifestyle or even their metabolism. Personally I do occasionally eat poultry or fish but I have found that on the whole vegetarianism suits my way of life. Not merely because I became troubled about the ethics of breeding animals for slaughter, but because it seems to bring me closer to the more natural way of living Yoga helps to enrich.

Certainly, I think it is true to say that the majority of vegetarians tend to be slimmer and look more healthy, probably because they take more time and care over the type of food they eat. If you decide to try alternative ways of eating, such as the vegetarian, vegan or macrobiotic diets, I would strongly recommend that you still balance your meals by using at least one of each of the essential food constituents. This will ensure you keep your meals healthy *and* interesting.

Yogis believe that some food contains life-force or *prana*. For them it is the quality not the quantity of food that is important. They aim to eat small quantities of food with a high life-force content. They argue that you should rise from a meal feeling 'light' and 'alive', not heavy and lethargic. It's a good, simple principle to work by in your day-to-day eating and meal-planning. And if you apply it, you'll rapidly find yourself making all sorts of discoveries. The over-cooked, the over-processed, the over-refined, the artificial – your own body will soon tell you how much of the precious life-force they actually contain.

The Natural Cookery recipes I've included at the end of this section (see pages 80 to 84) will hopefully give you further inspiration in your choice of health-giving meals, and the Natural Remedies which follow them indicate which foods help cure specific health problems.

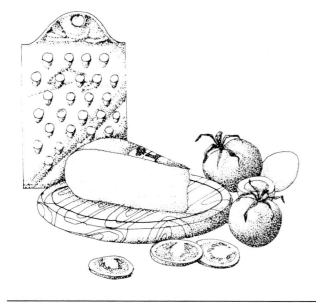

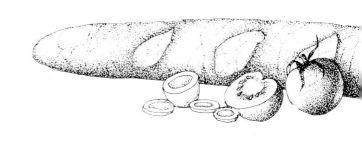

Preparing and eating your food

Once you've thought about the food you eat, it only makes sense to think about how you prepare it and even *how* you eat. The most carefully balanced meal is worthless if you gobble it up in the two minutes before you run for your morning train or while trying to persuade an irritable 3-year-old that his scrambled eggs aren't the most fiendish poison known to man.

Let's take the basic principles of preparation first:

1. Make sure all your food is fresh. Vitamin C, for example, is very short lived. Last week's lettuce won't rate highly and you should squeeze citrus fruits just before use.
2. Wash fruit and vegetables thoroughly. Remember some of the chemical sprays used in modern farming are poisonous. But don't be in a hurry to peel off the skins. They contain roughage, or fibre, which is essential to the elimination of waste products from the body, and in some cases most of the vitamin content as well.
3. Wherever possible, eat your fruits, vegetables and nuts raw. Once you start to cook, you start to destroy nutrients.
4. If cooking fruit or vegetables, keep the cooking time to a minimum. They should, wherever possible, maintain their crunchy texture when cooked.
5. The way you cook your food is very important. Steaming is one of the best ways of cooking. Other methods which have been practised for thousands of years and are still used by health-conscious cooks are baking in earthenware pots and slow casseroling. Chicken, fish and meat bricks are readily available, not only proving economical but also eliminating the need for fats, water or seasoning since the foods are cooked in their own juices. If you decide to boil food, use very little water and bring it to boiling point first. Reserve any remaining water for soups and stocks. Pans should be covered during cooking unless food is stir fried.
6. Seasoning should be added after food is cooked and here again kept to a minimum or the natural health-giving elements will be destroyed.

Now to the important point of how we eat. All our care in preparation will be lost if we bolt our food. Try to create a relaxed atmosphere over mealtimes. Food is a gift of nature and it should therefore be treated with reverence. If you are in a rush, then sit down to some fresh fruit or vegetables rather than a large meal which takes longer to digest properly. And remember always to chew your food thoroughly. You may think it ludicrous to mention this point, but check your own eating habits. Far too many of us get into the way of simply biting our food and swallowing it: we should be allowing the digestive juices a chance to begin breaking down our food even before it leaves the mouth.

Small wonder that constipation is such a common problem today. Yet beating this condition is really just a matter of common sense. A balanced diet based on the principles outlined above, good eating habits, and a sensible exercise programme are all that's required. And it's an effort that's well worth making. Not only will you feel so much happier and livelier. You'll really be fitter too. The human body was not designed to carry its waste products for any length of time. Rapid elimination is vitally important for your general health and well-being.

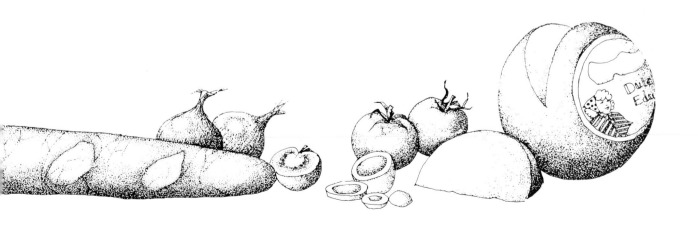

Cleansing diets and fasting

For thousands of years followers of Yoga have used the techniques of fasting. Many stories exist of yogis who have gone for days, even weeks, without food. Such feats have no relevance for most western followers: abstinence on this scale requires intensive and advanced training. Fasting is *not* the Yoga way to the slim, lithe body beautiful. However, it can play a part in your eating-for-health programme – either as the opener to your campaign or, probably more usefully, as a regular part of it. Its benefits as a cleansing technique are considerable.

Experiment for yourself. Try, say, setting one day a month aside for the Cleansing-Day Diet. But be sensible. Don't make it the day you've a heavy work schedule, the annual swimming gala or some big social event. You're not going to feel too energetic initially so it's best to choose a day when the pressure is off. As the months pass, you can, if you feel comfortable, try one of the 2-day Fruit Diets or the 2-day Fast. But always remember the purpose is to cleanse and purify the system. Coupled with a sensible eating programme and consistent exercise, these short periods of minimal eating or fasting can be enormously beneficial.

Cleansing-Day Diet

Metric/Imperial	American
Breakfast	
1 tomato	1 tomato
1 pear or peach	1 pear or peach
1 glass hot water with honey and lemon to taste	1 glass hot water with honey and lemon to taste
Mid-morning	
1 glass hot honey-and-lemon drink or lemon tea	1 glass hot honey-and-lemon drink or lemon tea
Lunch	
1 grated carrot	1 grated carrot
1 mashed banana or pear	1 mashed banana or pear
75 g/3 oz chopped white cabbage	$1\frac{3}{4}$ cups chopped white cabbage
above ingredients mixed with 1 (150 g/5·3 oz) carton natural yogurt or fresh orange juice	above ingredients mixed with $\frac{2}{3}$ cup of plain yogurt or fresh orange juice
1 glass iced water	1 glass iced water
Dinner	
as lunch	as lunch
1 glass hot honey-and-lemon drink	1 glass hot honey-and-lemon drink

Mixed Fruit Diet (2 days)

Metric/Imperial	American
Daily fruit allowance	
juice of 1 lemon	juice of 1 lemon
1 grapefruit	1 grapefruit
1 orange	1 orange
100 g/4 oz fresh or dried apricots	$\frac{2}{3}$ cup fresh or dried apricots
100 g/4 oz prunes or figs	$\frac{2}{3}$ cup prunes or figs
1 tablespoon honey	1 tablespoon honey
Prepare all ingredients and place in a bowl overnight	Prepare all ingredients and place in a bowl overnight
Breakfast	
50 g/2 oz wholegrain cereal with a little milk	1 cup wholegrain cereal with a little milk
1 teaspoon chopped almonds	1 teaspoon chopped almonds
lemon tea	lemon tea
Lunch	
half of prepared mixed fruit	half of prepared mixed fruit
50 g/2 oz Cheddar or cottage cheese	$\frac{1}{4}$ cup Cheddar or cottage cheese
lemon tea	lemon tea
Supper	
remainder of mixed fruit plus 1 teaspoon nuts	remainder of mixed fruit plus 1 teaspoon nuts
lemon tea	lemon tea

Repeat above menu on second day

Grape Diet (2 days)

Metric/Imperial	American
Breakfast	
$\frac{1}{2}$ grapefruit	$\frac{1}{2}$ grapefruit
100 g/4 oz green grapes	1 cup green grapes
Mid-morning	
50 g/2 oz green grapes	$\frac{1}{2}$ cup green grapes
Lunch	
$\frac{1}{2}$ grapefruit	$\frac{1}{2}$ grapefruit
100 g/4 oz black grapes	1 cup black grapes
Tea	
50 g/2 oz green grapes	$\frac{1}{2}$ cup green grapes
Dinner	
$\frac{1}{2}$ grapefruit	$\frac{1}{2}$ grapefruit
100 g/4 oz mixed black and green grapes	1 cup mixed black and green grapes

Peel each grape, so taking time to eat more slowly and making the meal feel much larger. Repeat menu on the second day. Drink natural mineral water. If you long for a hot drink, take decaffeinated coffee, with skimmed milk.

Fasting Diet (2 days)

Metric/Imperial	American
First Day	
1 glass warm, boiled water mixed with 1 teaspoon Epsom salts or an effervescent concentrated Vitamin C tablet	1 glass warm, boiled water mixed with 1 teaspoon Epsom salts or an effervescent concentrated Vitamin C tablet
300 ml/½ pint warm, boiled water	1¼ cups warm, boiled water
chilled water or apple juice	chilled water or apple juice

Drink warm water and salts/Vitamin C tablet on rising. Half an hour later drink the remaining warm water. During the rest of the day drink only small glasses of chilled fresh water or apple juice at 2–3 hourly intervals.

Second Day
Drink nothing until 6.00 pm, when you can celebrate with a glass of white wine or grape juice. Eat 4–6 bran biscuits or medium-sized slices of wholemeal toast during the day. These help to absorb the waste acids from the body when your liquid intake is reduced.

Return to your normal eating habits on the third day, remembering to eat little, slowly and often. Start the day with a glass of cold water.

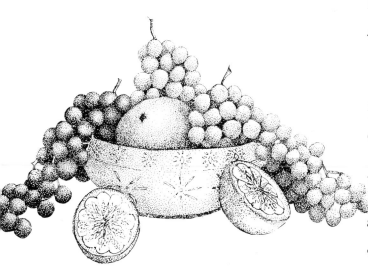

Weight control

Realism is the cornerstone of any weight-control programme. Whether your aim is weight gain or weight loss, the most important thing is to set yourself a personal, realistic target. The only time you should heed outside advice is if your doctor orders you to lose or gain weight.

Most of us, fortunately, don't have that problem. We simply feel we'd be healthier, more lively, more successful even, if our weight was a little more or a little less. Mostly we're comparing ourselves with other people – our friends or the models in magazines. We forget two very important points:

1. Each of us has our own sensible weight.
2. Any weight-control plan has got to be life-long.

Add these two points together and you're left in the exciting position of having to make all your own choices.

Plan your own schedule based on the principles of the Eating for Health programme outlined earlier, cutting down on the starchy, sugary foods (see page 75). Follow the exercises suggested in the earlier Weight Control section (see pages 47–51). And you'll be well on the way to the healthy outline that's right for you.

The following is a list of additional points and reminders which you'll find useful.

1. Consult your doctor or an expert in nutrition before embarking on your eating plan if you have any doubts about it.
2. Eat meals at regular times so that the body can establish its own harmonious rhythms. An overdose of food late at night when the body is less likely to need fuel is bound to turn to fat.
3. Try to have at least three balanced meals a day. Little and often is better than one heavy meal.
4. Before each meal, cleanse the system with a glass of mineral water or a piece of fruit or vegetable, e.g. pear, peach, sliced tomato or beetroot. Try to include at least one cleansing fruit or vegetable in your meal plan, e.g. leeks, lettuce, green vegetables or citrus fruit.
5. Cut down on the ritual of making cups of tea or coffee, which only swell the body.
6. Give yourself a rest from rich foods when you feel the need. Try a cleansing fruit diet or an occasional fast. (See page 78.)
7. It may take 6 months or more to achieve your ideal weight, but be patient. A realistic plan is much more likely to work and be maintained than any severe crash diet.
8. Couple your lifetime weight-control plan with regular daily exercise, preferably 3–4 hours after eating.
9. Don't make weight control an obsession. Keep your mind occupied with an interesting hobby.

Anorexia Nervosa

Recognizing early warning-signs and then finding expert help are the most effective ways of combating this alarming mental and physical disorder.

During my years as a teacher of Yoga more and more people suffering from anorexia have applied to us for help and advice. Thankfully, coupled with the guidance of a good psychiatrist or doctor, regular attendance at classes for relaxation, exercise and meditation has helped many sufferers.

Anorexia nervosa is a condition that causes immense distress not only to the sufferers but also to their families and friends. The typical victim is an intelligent young girl from an above average home; as yet the percentage of male sufferers is very small. The early signs are easy to detect: crash-dieting to the point of losing a third of the body weight, an aversion to carbohydrates, obsession with calories and weight, induced vomiting, depression and introversion, and deceit and cunning to hide the condition. Coupled with all this is the anorexic's inability to see what she or he is doing to the body. The thinner they become the more their conviction grows that they are fat. The condition leads to loss of periods, dry, brittle hair appearing on the body, fingernails growing weak, gum infections, epilepsy, kidney and stomach damage and severe depression.

Asking people why they become anorexic is like asking why they have nervous breakdowns. A family which puts a heavy emphasis on success, a broken home, boarding school, the fears and doubts of adolescence are some of the most common factors. The victim's attitude towards her/his parents is ambivalent: both seeking rejection by the refusal to eat and at the same time attention seeking. Food and eating come to symbolize love and affection, and become virtually the only means of communicating and expressing her/his feelings.

There are many theories about and proposed cures for anorexia: self-help, discipline, hypnosis, force-feeding, love, shock tactics, psycho and family therapy. The best cure, of course, is to persuade the person to want to get better. This is usually best achieved by the patient perseverance of a close friend or doctor.

The Yoga therapy for anorexics is to release the hidden tensions which initially caused the problem. All the exercises, meditations and Natural Cookery recipes mentioned in this book offer a new start to any anorexic sufferer. The programme for Depression and Anxiety (see page 24) is probably the best with which to begin recovery. But, like anyone else using the book, it's useful to spend some time first with the section on Breathing and Relaxation (see page 15).

Natural Cookery

Basic Muesli
Serves 6–8

This well-known breakfast cereal can also be used with fresh fruit salad or home-made ice cream, or as a topping for fruit crumbles.

Metric/Imperial	American
450 g/1 lb mixed grains, e.g. bran, wheatmeal, wheatgerm, oatflakes and maize	5 cups mixed grains, e.g. bran, wheatmeal, wheatgerm, oatflakes and maize
2 tablespoons skimmed milk powder	3 tablespoons skimmed milk powder
2 tablespoons chopped mixed nuts	3 tablespoons chopped mixed nuts
2 tablespoons raisins or sultanas	3 tablespoons seedless or seedless white raisins
2 tablespoons chopped dried apricots, apples or dates	3 tablespoons chopped dried apricots, apples or dates
1–2 tablespoons dark brown sugar	1–3 tablespoons dark brown sugar

1. Mix all the ingredients together and store in an airtight container.
2. Serve with hot or cold milk or water. Muesli is especially delicious served with yogurt and fresh chopped fruit.

Fresh Tomato Soup
Serves 4

Metric/Imperial	American
1 tablespoon vegetable oil	1 tablespoon vegetable oil
1 finely chopped onion	1 finely chopped onion
1 finely chopped carrot	1 finely chopped carrot
25 g/1 oz plain wholemeal flour	$\frac{1}{4}$ cup all-purpose wholemeal flour
600 ml/1 pint chicken or vegetable stock	$2\frac{1}{2}$ cups chicken or vegetable stock
1 bay leaf	1 bay leaf
675 g/1½ lb skinned and chopped fresh tomatoes	1½ lb skinned and chopped fresh tomatoes
1 teaspoon dark brown sugar	1 teaspoon dark brown sugar
pinch of rosemary	pinch of rosemary
salt and pepper	salt and pepper

1. Heat oil and gently saute onion and carrot for 5 minutes.
2. Remove the pan from the heat, add the flour, mixing it in and return to the heat, stirring continually. Cook for a minute and then stir in the stock, bay leaf, tomatoes, sugar and rosemary.
3. Bring to boiling point, then lower the heat, cover and simmer for 20–30 minutes.
4. Sieve or liquidize, and season. Serve hot or cold.

Basic Brown Bread

Like most new bread, this is best eaten the next day – to prevent indigestion. With a little practice, you'll soon be confidently making your own bread.

Metric/Imperial	American
3 teaspoons dried yeast	3 teaspoons active, dry yeast
2 teaspoons dark brown sugar	2 teaspoons dark brown sugar
1 crushed Vitamin C tablet	1 crushed Vitamin C tablet
450 ml/¾ pint warm water	2 scant cups warm water
25 g/1 oz vegetable margarine, melted	2 tablespoons vegetable margarine, melted
2 teaspoons ground sea salt	2 teaspoons ground sea salt
675 g/1½ lb plain wholemeal flour	6 cups all-purpose wholemeal flour

1. Cream the yeast, 1 teaspoon of sugar, and the Vitamin C tablet with 150 ml/¼ pint (US ⅔ cup) of warm water. Leave the mixture in a warm place for 10 minutes until frothy.
2. Stir the margarine, the remaining sugar, and the sea salt in the rest of the warm water. Add the yeast mixture.
3. Stir into the flour and mix to a firm dough. Knead on a lightly floured board for 10 minutes.
4. Divide dough in half and place in two warmed, greased 450-g/1-lb loaf tins. Seal both tins in a greased plastic bag.
5. Leave to rise for 30 minutes in a warm place.
6. Bake in the centre of a hot oven (230C, 450F, Gas Mark 8) for 30–40 minutes. Cool on a wire rack.

Oriental Salad
Serves 3–4

Metric/Imperial	American
½ Chinese cabbage	½ Chinese cabbage
1 green, red and/or yellow pepper	1 green, red and/or yellow pepper
Dressing	
1 tablespoon chopped stem ginger	1 tablespoon chopped preserved ginger
1 tablespoon dark brown sugar	1 tablespoon dark brown sugar
2 tablespoons tomato purée	3 tablespoons tomato paste
1 teaspoon chopped mint	1 teaspoon chopped mint
1 tablespoon vegetable oil (optional)	1 tablespoon vegetable oil (optional)
1 tablespoon cider vinegar	1 tablespoon cider vinegar
salt and pepper	salt and pepper

1. Chop the cabbage and peppers into bite-sized pieces.
2. Mix the remaining ingredients to form the dressing, seasoning to taste.
3. Toss vegetables and dressing together and serve chilled.

Cucumber Salad
Serves 4–6

This home-made yogurt dressing tastes really creamy without the sour taste of many manufactured yogurts. Without the cream, it will keep for a week in the refrigerator.

Metric/Imperial	American
Yogurt	
600 ml/1 pint long-life milk	2½ cups long-life milk
1 tablespoon natural yogurt	1 tablespoon plain yogurt
Salad	
600 ml/1 pint home-made natural yogurt	2½ cups home-made plain yogurt
150 ml/¼ pint double cream	⅔ cup heavy cream
1 medium cucumber	1 medium cucumber
2 cloves crushed or finely chopped garlic	2 cloves crushed or finely chopped garlic
2 tablespoons chopped mint and a few whole leaves for decoration	3 tablespoons chopped mint and a few whole leaves for decoration
paprika pepper	paprika pepper

To make the yogurt
1. Bring the milk to the boil and simmer for 2–3 minutes.
2. Cool to 41–3C, 106–7F, skim, and gently beat in the yogurt.
3. Pour the beaten milk into an earthenware bowl. Cover the top with foil and wrap the bowl in a small towel.
4. Store in a warm place for 8 hours. The yogurt is then ready for eating.

To make the salad
1. Gently whip the cream into the home-made yogurt.
2. Dice the cucumber, keeping a few thin slices for decoration.
3. Add the cucumber, garlic and mint to the yogurt and mix well. Season with paprika pepper to taste.
4. Chill and serve decorated with cucumber slices and mint leaves.

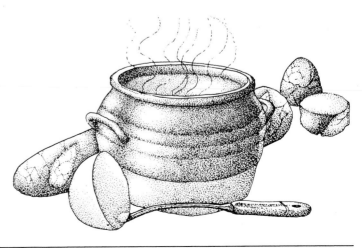

Corn and Herb Flan
Serves 4–6

The unique flavour of fresh or dried herbs makes this flan a light, tasty lunch dish.

Metric/Imperial	American
Herb Pastry Case (US Pie Shell)	
100 g/4 oz self-raising wholemeal flour	1 cup all-purpose wholemeal flour, sifted with baking powder
50 g/2 oz cornflour	scant ½ cup cornstarch
½ teaspoon ground sea salt	½ teaspoon ground sea salt
½ teaspoon chopped mixed fresh herbs or ¼ teaspoon mixed dried herbs	½ teaspoon chopped mixed fresh herbs or ¼ teaspoon mixed dried herbs
75 g/3 oz vegetable margarine	6 tablespoons vegetable margarine
water and/or 1 egg yolk for binding	water and/or 1 egg yolk for binding
Filling	
1 medium onion, chopped (optional)	1 medium onion, chopped (optional)
1 tablespoon vegetable oil	1 tablespoon vegetable oil
225 g/8 oz sweet corn	1½ cups corn
½ teaspoon chopped mixed fresh herbs or ¼ teaspoon mixed dried herbs	½ teaspoon chopped mixed fresh herbs or ¼ teaspoon mixed dried herbs
2 beaten eggs	2 beaten eggs
300 ml/½ pint single cream or natural yogurt	1½ cups light cream or plain yogurt
salt and pepper	salt and pepper
75 g/3 oz grated cheese	¾ cup grated cheese

To make the case (US shell)
1. Place the flour, cornflour (US cornstarch), sea salt and herbs in a bowl and rub in the margarine until the mixture looks like fine breadcrumbs.
2. Bind with enough water and/or the egg yolk to make a firm dough.
3. Roll out the pastry and line a 20-cm/8-inch flan tin (US pie pan). Prick the sides and base with a fork.
4. Bake blind in a moderately hot oven (200C, 400F, Gas Mark 6) for 10 minutes.

To make the filling
1. Heat the oil and cook the onion until transparent. Drain on absorbent paper.
2. Mix the onion, sweet corn (US corn), herbs, egg and cream or yogurt together and season.
3. Pour the mixture into the pre-cooked flan case (US shell) and top with the grated cheese.
4. Reduce the oven temperature slightly (190C, 375F, Gas Mark 5) and bake in the centre of the oven for 20–25 minutes.

Leek Gougère
Serves 4

This simple French recipe can be varied to include any savoury filling. The flan case is light with the texture of choux pastry and the dish should be served straight from the oven. The results always reap compliments.

Metric/Imperial	American
450 g/1 lb leeks, carefully washed and chopped into 5-cm/2-inch pieces	1 lb leeks, carefully washed and chopped into 2-inch pieces
100 g/4 oz margarine	½ cup margarine
200 g/7 oz plain wholemeal flour	1¾ cups all-purpose wholemeal flour
4 eggs	4 eggs
50 g/2 oz butter	4 tablespoons butter
300 ml/½ pint milk	1½ cups milk
¼ teaspoon French mustard	¼ teaspoon French mustard
50 g/2 oz grated Gruyère cheese	½ cup grated Gruyère cheese
salt and pepper	salt and pepper

1. Cook the leeks in boiling water for approximately 5 minutes or until tender.
2. Drain the water into a measuring jug and make up to 300 ml/½ pint (US 1¼ cups). Pour the water into another pan and add the margarine. Heat gently until the margarine melts and then return to boiling point.
3. Remove the pan from the heat and beat in 175 g/6 oz (US 1½ cups) flour. Add ½ teaspoon of salt.
4. Beat in the eggs, one at a time.
5. Spread ⅔ of the mixture over the base of a greased 20-cm/8-inch flan tin (US pie pan). Pipe or spoon the remainder around the edge of the base to make a flan case (US pie shell).
6. Melt the butter over a low heat and stir in the remaining flour. Cook for a minute and then add the milk and bring to the boil, stirring continuously. Return the sauce to the heat, still stirring, and add the mustard and the cooked leeks. Season to taste.
7. Spoon the leeks and their sauce onto the flan case and sprinkle the top with the cheese.
8. Bake in a moderately hot oven (200C, 400F, Gas Mark 6) for 35–40 minutes.

Easy Fish Bake
Serves 4

This is the simplest fish bake I know, and the results are delicious.

Metric/Imperial	American
450 g/1 lb filleted cod or halibut	1 lb filleted cod or halibut
150 ml/¼ pint milk	⅔ cup milk
25 g/1 oz vegetable margarine	2 tablespoons vegetable margarine
salt and pepper	salt and pepper
Topping	
100 g/4 oz fresh wholemeal breadcrumbs	2 cups fresh, soft wholemeal breadcrumbs
100 g/4 oz Cheddar cheese with onion and chives, grated	½ cup Cheddar cheese with onion and chives, grated
chopped parsley	chopped parsley
wedges of lemon for decoration	wedges of lemon for decoration

1. Wash the fish pieces, skin and place in a greased ovenproof dish. Cover with the milk and dot with margarine. Add seasoning.
2. Bake in a moderate oven (180C, 350F, Gas Mark 4) for 15 minutes.
3. Mix the breadcrumbs, cheese and most of the parsley together and sprinkle over the baked fish. Return to the oven for another 30 minutes, until the topping is golden brown.
4. Decorate with the remainder of the parsley and wedges of lemon, and serve hot with tomato or cucumber salad.

Summer Pudding
Serves 4–6

This favourite pudding can be made all the year round, using a mixture of the fruits in season or dried fruit which has been soaked overnight and lightly poached in orange juice.

Metric/Imperial	American
900g/2 lb mixed fresh fruit, such as black and red currants, raspberries, strawberries, blackberries, apples, cherries, pears, pineapple, guavas, apricots, gooseberries or peaches	2 lb mixed fresh fruit, such as black and red currants, raspberries, strawberries, blackberries, apples, pears, pineapple, guavas, apricots, gooseberries or peaches
75–100 g/3–4 oz dark brown sugar or honey	6–8 tablespoon dark brown sugar or honey
about 8 (1-cm/½-inch thick) slices of bread (crusts removed) or fruit loaf	about 8 (½-inch) slices of bread (crusts removed) or fruit loaf
fruit leaves for decoration (optional)	fruit leaves for decoration (optional)

1. Simmer gently all but 100 g/4 oz (US 1 cup) of the fruits with the sugar or honey for 5 minutes or until tender.
2. Line a 900-ml/1½-pint (US 2-pint) greased pudding basin (US mold) or souffle dish with the slices of bread, or fruit loaf, reserving several slices for the top.
3. Strain the fruit and spoon it into the lined basin. Keep the strained juice for last-minute repairs. Cover the top of the basin with the remaining slices of bread or fruit loaf.
4. Place a plate on top of the basin, press it down with a heavy weight, and chill overnight.
5. Take the pudding out of the mould by removing the plate, gently easing the sides away from the basin with a knife, placing a serving dish on top of the basin and turning the basin upside down.
6. Carefully pour the strained juice over the bread or fruit loaf just before serving.
7. Decorate with the remaining fruits and seasonal leaves and serve.

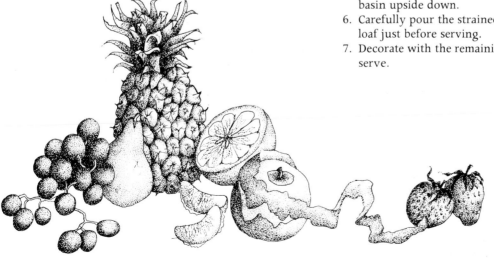

Hot Lemon Delicious
Serves 4–6

Metric/Imperial	American
grated rind and juice of 1 lemon	grated rind and juice of 1 lemon
50 g/2 oz butter	4 tablespoons butter
100 g/4 oz dark brown sugar or honey	$\frac{1}{2}$ cup dark brown sugar or honey
2 eggs	2 eggs
50 g/2 oz self-raising wholemeal flour	$\frac{1}{2}$ cup all-purpose wholemeal flour sifted with baking powder
300 ml/$\frac{1}{2}$ pint milk	$1\frac{1}{4}$ cups milk

1. Cream the lemon rind, butter and sugar together until soft.
2. Separate the egg yolks and whites. Add the beaten egg yolks and a little flour to the butter and sugar mixture and stir well.
3. Gradually stir in the milk, lemon juice and remaining flour, a little at a time of each ingredient in turn.
4. Beat the egg whites until stiff, and fold evenly into the mixture.
5. Pour into a greased 900-ml/1$\frac{1}{2}$ pint (US 1$\frac{3}{4}$ pint) ovenproof bowl and bake in a moderately hot oven (180C, 350F, Gas Mark 4) for 40–50 minutes.

Fruity Flapjacks

Children love making these biscuits. Full of natural goodness and flavoured with dried fruit, they have a delicious moist texture. You can vary the recipe by experimenting with your own combinations of dried ingredients.

Metric/Imperial	American
100 g/4 oz vegetable margarine	$\frac{1}{2}$ cup vegetable margarine
1 tablespoon dark brown sugar	1 tablespoon dark brown sugar
3 tablespoons orange marmalade	scant $\frac{1}{4}$ cup orange marmalade
75 g/3 oz rolled oats	$\frac{3}{4}$ cup rolled oats
75 g/3 oz ground almonds	$\frac{3}{4}$ cup ground almonds
75 g/3 oz dessicated coconut	$\frac{3}{4}$ cup dessicated coconut
50–75 g/2–3 oz stem ginger or any other dried fruit	$\frac{1}{2}$ cup stem ginger or any other dried fruit

1. Melt the margarine, sugar and marmalade together.
2. Remove the pan from the heat and add all the other ingredients, mixing them thoroughly.
3. Spread over the base of a 20-cm/8-inch greased cake tin.
4. Bake in a moderately hot oven (190C, 375F, Gas Mark 5) for 15–20 minutes.
5. Leave to cool slightly, cut into slices, and remove from the tin when cold.

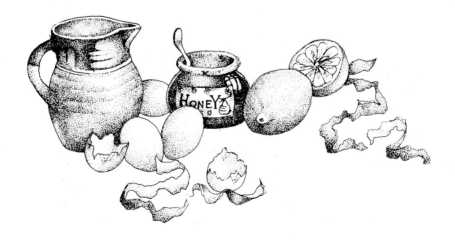

Natural remedies

Include the suggested foods for your ailment in a balanced diet and you will get relief from, and even cure, your problem.
Note The natural oils are used for external massage.

Overwork Apricots, currants, bananas, nuts, lemons, oranges, peppers, spinach, soya beans, lettuce, honey. Herb tea: camomile.

Headache and Migraine Cabbage juice, apple juice, beetroot, rice, rye, potatoes, decaffeinated coffee. Herb teas: mint, camomile, lemon balm. *Avoid* refined products (such as white flour, cereal and sugar), stimulants (such as tea, coffee, alcohol and chocolate), and dairy products (such as cheese and milk). Keep meals simple and follow the philosophy that fresh is best. Natural mineral water taken before every meal is another known cure.

Depression and Anxiety Almonds, avocados, peanuts, corn oil, mushrooms.

High Blood Pressure Carrots, citrus fruits, blackcurrants, grapes, parsley, garlic, radishes, cucumber, tomatoes. Herb tea: jasmine.

Low Blood Pressure Dates, figs, currants, leeks, onions, nuts, soya beans.

Weak Heart Vegetable and fruit juices, parsley, garlic. Herb teas: hawthorn, rosemary.

Insomnia Apples, carrots, cabbage, parsley, watermelon, lettuce. Herb teas. Bath oils: orange blossom, sandlewood.

Infertility Ginseng with Vitamin E, bonemeal, beans, rice, watercress, lettuce, peas.

Pregnancy As for **Infertility**, plus all fresh fruit and vegetables, wheat germ, yeast, soya flour, liver, kidneys, grapefruit, pears, tomatoes.

Menstrual Disorders All green vegetables, beetroot, lettuce, fennel, figs, parsley, grapes. Herb teas.

Sinus Congestion Leeks, onions, tomatoes, garlic, lettuce, oranges, lemons, grapes, honey, clear vegetable soups including cabbage and carrots, parsley, potatoes baked in their jackets, salads. Herb teas. Inhale the steam from a bowl of boiling water, having first covered the head with a towel. *Avoid* dairy products, particularly milk.

Colds and Flu Vegetable juices and soups, garlic, onions, oranges, lemons, grapefruit, blackcurrants. Herb teas: camomile, peppermint, lemon balm, sage. Oils of eucalyptus, camphor, rosemary.

Sore Throats Try a glass of warm water with lemon and honey or gargle with boiled water and sea-salt or sea water.

Chilblains Boil 250 g/9 oz (US 2$\frac{1}{4}$ cups) chopped celery stalks in 1 litre/1$\frac{3}{4}$ pints (US 4$\frac{1}{4}$ cups) water. Cool and immerse hands and feet in strained juice for 5 minutes.

Asthma and Bronchitis Mix one part castor oil to two parts honey and take one teaspoon of the mixture morning and night. Apples, apricots, cabbage, cherries, figs, peaches, lemons, tangerines, nectarines, oranges, honey. Herb tea: peppermint.

Back Ache Warm mustard baths, plenty of fresh fruit and vegetables. *Avoid* stimulants, such as tea and coffee or alcohol.

Constipation Start your day with one of the following: half a grapefruit; 125 g/4 oz (US 1 cup) prunes, peaches, figs or pears, fresh or dried and soaked overnight; 2 tomatoes and 1 glass of mineral water; 1 fresh pear and 75 g/2 tablespoons bran soaked in hot water; or two over-ripe bananas. For main meals always include at least one of the cleansing fruits or vegetables, i.e. leeks, tomatoes, beetroot, rhubarb, grapes, onions, carrots, watercress. Cooked rice in last meal of day is also helpful. *Avoid* dairy products and refined foods (see **Headache and Migraine**).

Diarrhoea Unripe bananas, barley, kale, mushrooms, oranges, parsnips, potatoes, rice, soya beans, tapioca, spinach, cabbage juice, nettles, blueberries, raspberries.

Acne Take a glass of mineral water before each meal. Sunlight and fresh air, brewer's yeast, cabbage, tomatoes, tomato juice, pears, grapefruit, alfalfa, cress. Herb teas: dandelion, nettle. Oils of camphor, sandlewood. *Avoid* animal by-products: goat's milk is preferable.

Skin Burns Skin of potato, cabbage (cut side), banana. Oils of camphor, camomile, rosemary.

Overweight As for **Constipation**.

Ageing Limbs Apricots, dates, ginseng, cabbage, garlic, pineapples, seaweed, honey, liver. Herb tea: elder flower.

Baldness Gently massage the whole scalp with witch hazel before retiring to bed. Leave for a few minutes and then massage with warm olive oil. Try to leave the oil on overnight before removing with a mild shampoo.

Deafness Cabbage, apples, carrots, cauliflowers, turnips, lettuce, in fact all crunchy fruit or vegetables, which help to exercise the inner-ear muscles.

Weak Eyesight Apricots, carrots, coconut, dandelions, grapefruit, onions, prunes, watercress, fish, liver, ginseng with Vitamin E.

Keeping Warm Barley, lentils, oats, rice, wholemeal flour and by-products, potatoes, citrus fruits, vegetable extract, honey, milk, yogurt, vegetable broths and oils.

Multiple Sclerosis All fresh fruit and vegetables, especially grapes, apricots, pears, tomatoes, mangoes, pineapple.

Arthritis Asparagus, artichokes, beans, garlic, carrots, cucumbers, grapefruit, melons, parsley, pineapples, pomegranates, spinach. Herb teas. Oil of rosemary.

Rheumatism Fruit and vegetable juices, Vitamin B^{12} supplement, carrots, celery, tomatoes, grapes, vegetable oils, nuts, parsley, cabbage, coconut. *Avoid* meat, eggs, tea, coffee, acid fruits, such as apples and oranges.

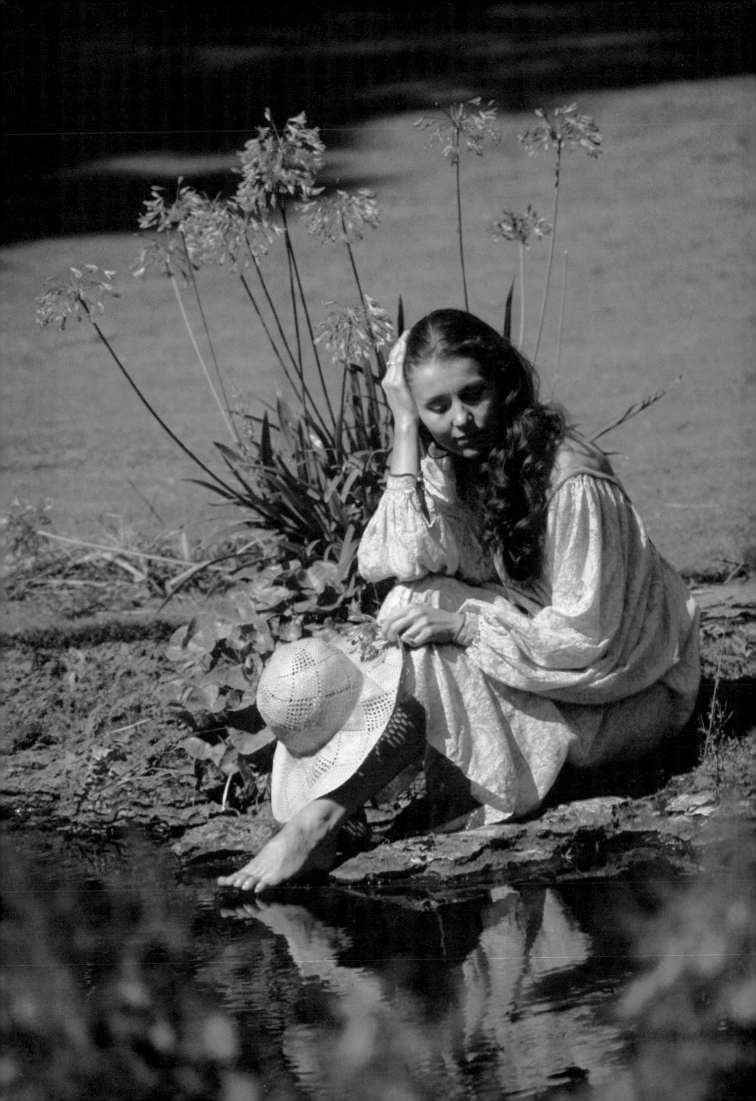

Meditation

Yoga is not simply about exercises, about the physical relief of physical ailments. It is about the attainment of a deep peace, an inner calm that stems from achieving a harmony between your mind and your body, your self and the world around you. The ideal is to be harmoniously balanced, centred, happy, calm and freely creative.

It is essential, if you are going to study Yoga at all, that you explore it as a way to meditation. Don't let the idea of meditation put you off; it's not a difficult, remote kind of mental gymnastics, but a practical way of calming your spirit, of finding the peace and beauty that is inside you. Learning to meditate with Yoga can mean finding a peace, a relaxation, more complete than you have known for years.

Meditation is the science of stilling and controlling the mind. Most people would want to meditate if they understood its value and experienced its beneficial effects. What achievement could be more purposeful and useful than the harnessing of the qualities of peace, love, joy, power and wisdom?

Concentrating to learn

People who become completely absorbed by their work or hobby are practising a form of meditation or concentration without tension. For a slip-second time becomes nothing and everything is one: only later do they become aware of what has happened.

Meditation utilizes concentration in its highest form. Concentration consists of freeing the attention from distractions and of focusing on a chosen thought or object. For many of us living in the rush of daily life there seems little enough time to concentrate on the things we really wish to do. But with guidance we can all enjoy the fruits of meditation and find a deeper awareness that improves not only superficial concentration but also our understanding of the real meaning of life.

To achieve pure concentration we need periods of disciplined silence. One of the best ways to start is to impose short periods of silence on yourself, perhaps over mealtimes. This not only slows you down but makes you more aware of the way you breathe, the way you move. In fact every sense is heightened through silent concentration.

To take what you've learned further, you must find a special place where you can go to be quiet. Somewhere you can retreat without fear or guilt. Go with the thankful knowledge that here you can enjoy being yourself. Here it does not matter whether you are bad tempered, greedy, envious, fat or thin. Here you have no one to impress or please. There is no need to communicate. You are now completely free to enjoy your own thoughts.

As always, the first step is to clear away all the tensions of your life. Remembering all you learned in the Breathing and Relaxation section (see page 15), relax in the Resting Pose and breathe the Complete Breath to your own natural rhythm.

Gently close your eyes, and let your physical tensions ripple away. Feel your cool breath soothing the back of your throat, chest and lungs.

> Breathe in peace; breathe out turmoil.
> Breathe in truth; breathe out lies.
> Breathe in strength; breathe out weakness.
> Breathe in love; breathe out love.

Now you are ready to practise the deep relaxation which will lead you into slip-second meditation. The technique you are going to use differs from that you learned in the Breathing and Relaxation section in its intensity rather than any essential characteristics. Once again you lead your consciousness through the different parts of the body but this time you break down the various limbs, etc. into even smaller centres of interest with the result that the effects are greatly heightened.

Deep relaxation Simply allow your mind to become aware of the different parts of your body. Think of each part in turn, relaxing any physical tension and visualizing it as being totally healthy and full of vitality. Try not to strain your concentration, and pause for a brief moment as you dwell upon each part.

Begin, for example, with the right side of your body. Think of your right hand: the thumb, the first finger, the second, the third, the fourth. Become aware of your palm, the wrist, the elbow, the shoulder, the armpit, the right side of your waist, the right hip, the thigh, the kneecap, the calf muscle, the ankle, the heel, the sole of the right foot, the big toe, the second toe, the third toe, the fourth toe, the fifth toe. Then go on to the left side of the body, to your back, and to your front, starting at the top of your head and working downwards from the forehead to the eyebrows (taken separately) and so on.

Once you've completed this total breakdown and concentration upon individual parts of the body, begin the process of uniting it in heightened awareness. Think of the whole of your right leg, the whole of your left leg, both legs, the whole of the left arm, the right arm, both arms, the spine, the shoulder blades, the buttocks, the whole of the back, and so on.

Though sleep will be a temptation, try to remain totally aware. Your whole body rests very still on the floor. See your body lying perfectly still and peacefully on the floor in this particular room. . . .

Become aware of your breath. Feel its flow in and out of your lungs. Do not try to change the rhythm. Let it take its own natural, healthy pattern. Immerse yourself totally in that pattern. Now concentrate your awareness on the movement of your navel. It rises and falls very slightly with each breath. Begin mentally counting from 15 to 1 in time to your breathing:

15 *inhale* as navel rises
14 *exhale* as navel falls
13 *inhale* as navel rises. . . .

If you make a mistake, go back and start again.

Stop counting and become aware of your chest expanding and relaxing. After a few breaths, turn your concentration to your throat. Feel the cool breath of inhalation and the warm breath of exhalation. Now think about the breath moving in and out of your nostrils. . . .

Slip-second meditation Detach your mind from your family: think of them and slowly, one by one, detach yourself from them. Detach your mind from your friends: think of them and slowly detach. Detach from your work and chores. Hear no particular sound. Have no particular thought. Simply rest and enjoy being yourself.

The slip-second formula is best practised at least once every day, preferably at the same time of day. Once the technique is perfected, you will find you are able totally to detach from your surroundings for very brief moments of time. Time itself will seem to stand still and everything will join together in complete, harmonious peace.

Like so many of the benefits of Yoga, the effects of this exercise are not necessarily evident as you practise. The revitalizing of the mind and body can show itself in the form of healthy energy either later in the day or even the following day.

Candle meditation You're ready now to begin another exercise in concentration. It's a technique that's sometimes called inner visualization, and it involves a relaxed concentration upon a chosen object. A tradition has grown up of using a candle flame for this exercise but in fact almost any small object could be used. The purpose of the exercise is to increase calmness and mental altertness by simply turning the mind inwards towards the sources of energy and thus prepare for the next stage of meditation.

1. Sit comfortably with the spine erect but not rigid.
2. Place a lighted candle at eye level and an arm's length away.
3. Relax for a few minutes, breathing the Complete Breath to your natural rhythm and gently closing your eyes.
4. Open your eyes and concentrate on the top of the candle flame for a few Complete Breaths. Absorb its light, warmth, shape and colour.
5. Gently close your eyes and in your mind's eye recall every feature of the flame, holding the image in your imagination. Every time your mind wanders, open your eyes and renew your impression of the flame so that it becomes more vividly imprinted on your imagination once you reclose your eyes.
6. When you are able to think only of the flame, you are ready to move onto the next stage.

Now try another exercise in concentration. Using your imagination, your intellect, your emotions and your senses, try to visualize some scene or natural landscape: snowcapped mountains, birds flying across a sunset, waves breaking on a deserted shore. . . .

You are what you think

Inner visualization isn't merely a mental trick to aid concentration. By internalizing that candle flame or imagining some natural landscape you've been schooling your imagination, making it work *for* you rather than against you. Now let's take that technique a stage further. By directing the imagination with positive thinking we can create an emotional climate which enhances our general health – mental, physical and spiritual. Eating wholesome food creates healthy bodies. In the same way, as you think in your heart, so you are.

All through life your conscious mind has picked up good and bad thoughts and impressions, which have taken root in your subconscious. Every kind of success or failure in life is to a large extent the result of the thoughts and ideas which you have given dominance in your mind. If negative impressions have become firmly fixed, a determined effort is needed to replace them. New, positive impressions must be built up to such a degree that the old ones no longer have any power. Believe that this is possible because it is never too late to master the whole pattern of your life.

The fearful 'I can't' takes priority over the courageous 'I can' unless you take yourself in hand. In the face of adversity you can win through or give in. The issue of success or failure is obviously determined by your attitude of mind. There is no luck or chance in this: it is the logic of cause and effect. By visualizing something better in yourself than you have so far achieved and by giving such thoughts reality through your actions, you will soon not only influence your circumstances but also control your stress and improve your health.

The positive way to practical meditation

The simplest way to start daily meditation is to have a thought for the day, i.e. a simple maxim to hold in your mind as you go about the business of living. Here are some I have found useful:

My kingdom is within me.

I believe that I am the architect of my own fate. I will be master of my circumstances, not their slave.

The morrow will bring new strength, new hopes, new opportunities and new beginnings.

I will conquer all obstacles and turn them into opportunities.

I will not waste my mental energies in useless worry.

One minute of anger is 60 seconds of unhappiness and perhaps hours of remorse.

I will maintain perfect health.
I will become positive and dynamic.
I will be true to myself.

Many students find it helpful at first to read written meditations. To be told that the power to face every challenge lies within themselves is for some stricken with anxiety and self-doubt very hard to believe and to others positively daunting. For this reason I have decided to conclude with several examples of positive meditation.

Slowing down Slow down and ease the pounding of your heart by the quieting of your mind. Steady your hurried pace with a vision of eternity. Break the tension of your nerves and moods with soothing music or the power of sleep. Teach yourself the art of taking minute meditations, of slowing down to enjoy the beauty of a flower or bird, to chat to a friend, pat a dog or cat, or read a few lines from a good book or a poem. Remind yourself that there is more to life than the measuring of speed. Look into the branches of a tree and know that it is green and strong because it grew slowly and well. Send your own roots down into the soil of life's enduring values.

Stilling the mind with peace You need time to be still, to unwind. You may feel as you read this that stillness is the last thing you need. What you want is something to make you spring into life and action. But the most invigorating thing you can do at any time – on rising, halfway through your day, or before you go to bed – is to take a few minutes just to be still, to say to your body, to your mind, emotions, thoughts and feelings,

> Be still: peace is here.

You have great reserves of strength and power. In stillness you renew your energy, rebuild your body, reshape your thoughts, and calm your emotions.

At times your anxieties seem so great that you find it difficult to be still. Take a break from what you are doing or thinking and say the single word,

> Peace

Take a deep breath and say quietly to yourself or think,

> I am still and peaceful.

Then, as you consciously let the breath go, a sense of peace will come over you. You will have the assurance that the things that caused you concern are in the care and keeping of your inner strength. You will feel an inner peace growing; you will feel relaxed within yourself.

In simple stillness your whole being comes into harmony with your inner strength. The days get better, the worries, cares, pressures and demands slip away as you release yourself into being still.

> Harmony be in my waking.
> Harmony be in my thinking.
> Harmony be in my speaking.
> Harmony be in my sleeping.

Enjoying the flow of life Having learnt the art of deep relaxation, you can appreciate the natural rhythm of your body as you live life in a relaxed yet positive way.

Life flows as surely and constantly as a great river. So long as we move with it the current is strong and true to support us. It lends us energy as it carries us along. But when we dam the flow, block up the current of energy, the water becomes stagnant and, rather than being supported by life, we risk the poison of misdirected energies.

We must learn to allow changes both in ourselves and others. It is wrong to hold people to you when the current begins to carry them away. One of you will be stifled or hurt. You must let go and be open to new influences, new positive energies. As your life moves on and you see growth and change in yourself and people you know and love, allow yourselves to be free to follow the natural current of life.

There is no sin in utilizing emotions, people or objects for good until the time comes to change. Clinging to people and objects can only spoil them. Hoarding can be destructive. Open your heart and mind to the forces of good that are bound to come into your life, but be willing to let them go and to accept the new forces for good which may take their place.

Do not weep over failure or censure others for disappointing you. One of the secrets of life is to expect nothing. Good and bad experiences are all part of the current and flow of life, part of the changing pattern that is proof you are alive. Let the river of life flow through the triangle of your body, mind, and spirit.

Finding inner strength You do not have to wait until some indefinite future to realise your inner strength. You do not have to wait until you are out of your difficulty or the disharmony in which you find yourself. Your inner strength is with you now, right where you are. Every minute of your existence you live and move and have your being in this natural strength, and the fullness of love, power, and peace is with you.

When the temptation comes to run away from life and from

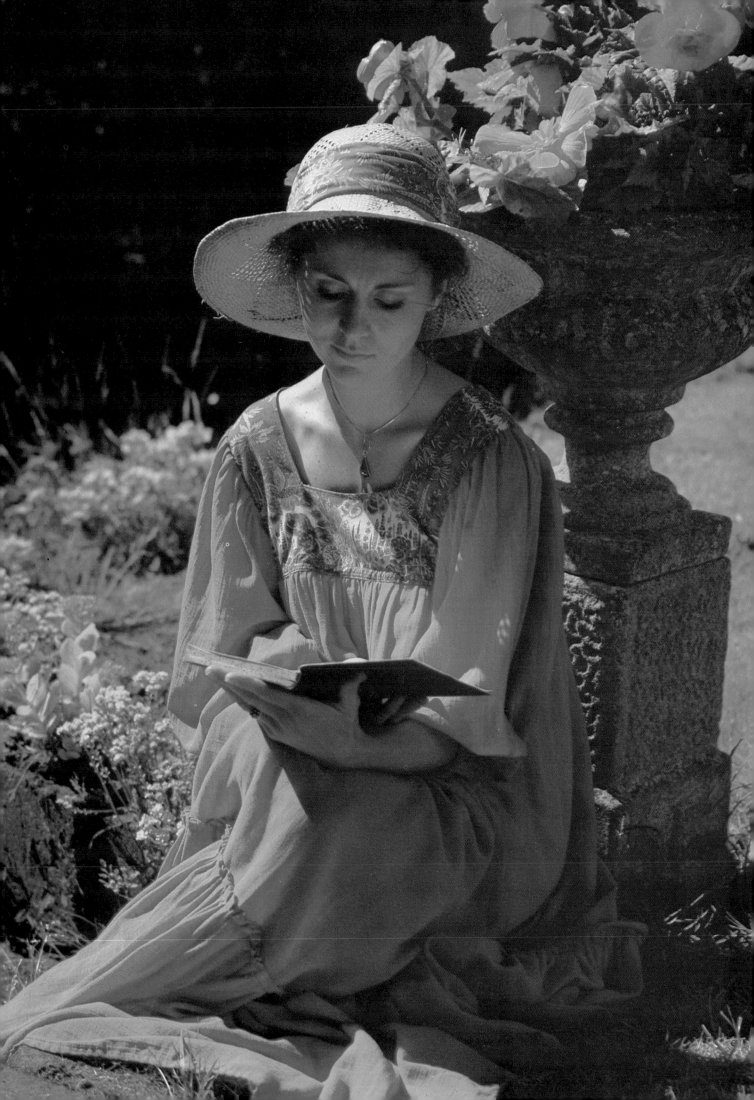

distressing circumstances, just simply stop, become still and ask yourself:

Why am I afraid when the strength is within, waiting for me to trust its power?

Keep your thoughts quietly on the strength within and the mists of negation will disperse. Peace will flow into your heart and assure you that all is well. Constantly practise thinking healing thoughts and you will be filled with the joy of living. And with it will come new vitality, new confidence, and new courage. You will go forward strengthened in mind and body. All of life will be brighter in your eyes. Your understanding will be quickened, your abilities expanded. At any hour of the day or night just call upon the power of the strength within you.

Overcoming fear and worry These are times of great change, both in world affairs and in the lives of individuals. However, they offer no cause for fear or insecurity to the student of meditation, whose faith is placed in the power of the spirit within. No matter what world or personal circumstances are, you will always find that in the way of meditation your life is harmonious.

Even in periods of great unrest you are always in touch with the source of goodness within your being. Look to your inner spirit for guidance and enlightenment by simply sitting still and peaceful for a short time each day. Simply try to be still and peaceful and know that your spirit is with you and that its wonderful power is yours. Meditate very quietly in faith and confidence. You know that your inner strength is greater than all your problems and that you have the power to reject as a denial of truth every negative, destructive thought: unsupported by your thoughts all appearances such as these simply vanish. No matter how real and distressing any situation facing you may appear to be, remember that as you are, still and peaceful, your power within is greater.

Gradually you will begin to consider many of your problems superficial and unnecessary. You will become convinced that they are magnified by your own thoughts. Now, in this clearer state of mind, you can rest from the pressures of your life for short intervals, knowing that when you return to the outside world your inner sanctuary will give you the strength you need to be able to cope with, and in many cases solve, life's challenges. Within us all is the power to face every challenge with a confident and cheerful heart, the power to meet and overcome every obstacle, the power to live triumphantly and successfully.

You will find you are led day by day into security, and in peace you will pass through any complications that may arise in your life. You will, with practice, learn that there is no need to fear changes. You will not be anxious about your affairs but secure in the knowledge that all problems pass and that you are working towards the establishment of inner peace. There is no problem that can defeat the supreme

power of your own spirit. Think to yourself:

Love is within me, around me, protecting me. I will banish the gloom of fear that shuts out the guiding light and makes me stumble into error.

Love is the great power that binds and joins in harmony the universe and everything in it. It is often difficult to express love in a situation in which your pride has been hurt, your security threatened, your trust betrayed. As soon as possible go still and become peaceful, affirming,

I am full of peace and harmony.

Then you will find it is love that harmonizes. It is love that brings a sense of oneness with your own innermost life. It is love that brings true awareness of inner peace and clears the mind so that the way ahead can be seen very clearly.

Index

Figures in **bold** indicate illustrated exercises.